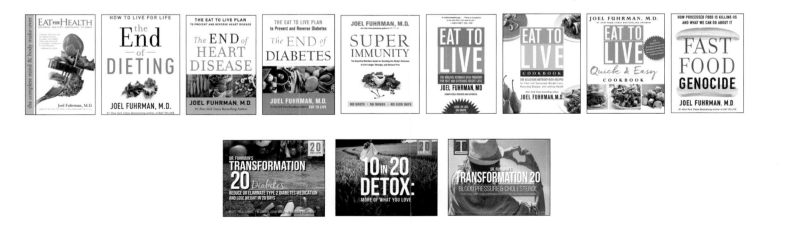

DR. FUHRMAN'S
100 BEST FOODS
FOR HEALTH AND LONGEVITY

Joel Fuhrman, M.D.

Published by:
Gift of Health Press

ghp

C O N T E N T S

of the 100 Best Foods for Health and Longevity.

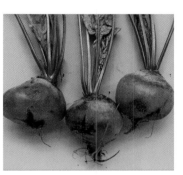
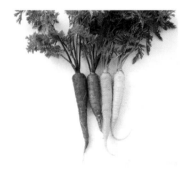
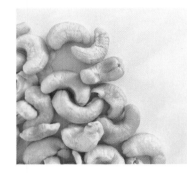
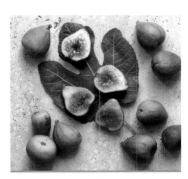

"It is not enough to know what I have for breakfast or lunch; rather, it is more important to find out why I focus my diet on these 100 particular foods."

59
GOJI BERRIES
Goji berries have been used for thousands of years as both a food and medicinal herb to treat diabetes and improve eyesight.

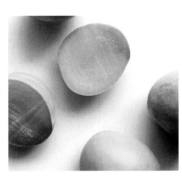

75
MANGO
Mangoes contain an abundance of vitamins, carotenoids, fiber, and phytochemicals.

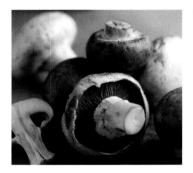

79
MUSHROOMS
Although they don't always get the respect they deserve, mushrooms are a superfood.

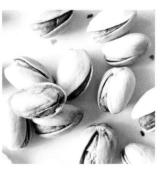

96
PISTACHIOS
Pistachios have the highest plant sterol content of all nuts, which helps to lower cholesterol levels.

118
SWISS CHARD
Swiss chard is one of the richest sources of carotenoids which help to preserve eye health and prevent age-related Macular Degeneration.

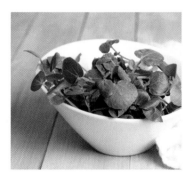

124
WATERCRESS
One of the healthiest foods in the world, everyone will get lifespan benefits from adding watercress to their diet.

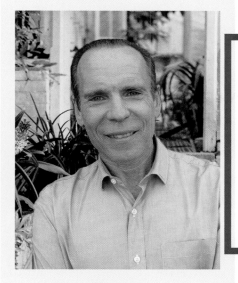

100 FOODS FOR 100 YEARS

To help you make the best choices when deciding what to eat, I created this index of the 100 Best Foods for Health and Longevity. There are many amazing benefits to eating the right foods. By learning about the special health benefits of individual superfoods, I am sure that you will be more inclined to make these nutrient-dense foods a central part of your diet.

The 100 Best Foods listed here are certainly not the only healthy foods out there, but they are the most commonly available ones. I'm sure there are many more nutrient-dense whole foods, especially in remote areas. However, these 100 foods form the basis of the healthiest diet available in most areas.

In my nutrition-oriented medical practice, I have watched thousands of patients lose excess weight permanently, and recover from serious diseases which were thought to be irreversible and lifelong. I have found that the right portfolio of protective foods, shown to prevent cancer and extend human lifespan, also possesses tremendous therapeutic potential to reverse diseases including diabetes, heart disease, migraines, autoimmune illnesses, and even some early-stage cancers.

Optimal health begins with nutrient-rich foods.

As a society, we consume many foods that have zero nutritional value, such as commercial baked goods, luncheon meats, fried foods, ice cream, soda, and white flour products.

These foods are highly addictive and dangerous, and their spread throughout the world has led to historically high rates of obesity, heart disease and type 2 diabetes.

The 100 whole plant foods listed here promote superior health and increase vitality.

The vitamins, minerals and phytochemicals in a nutrient-dense, plant-rich diet fuel the proper functioning of our immune system, and enable the detox and repair mechanisms of our cells to function optimally. This sets the stage not only for protection from chronic disease, but also for disease reversal. In addition, most whole plant foods are naturally low in calories and high in fiber, a perk for those seeking to lose weight.

Nutritional excellence also reduces appetite, removes food cravings and abnormal hunger signals, therby making it less likely to overeat (and can make it difficult to overconsume calories.) It is the most powerful and effective way to lose weight, and to maintain a healthy weight forever.

The more nutrient-dense food you consume, the more you satisfy your body with fewer calories, and the less you will crave fattening, high-calorie foods.

It really is that simple.

It is my hope that the knowledge you learn here will influence your decisions about which foods to include in your daily diet. For instance, you'll discover that cruciferous vegetables like broccoli, cauliflower, kale, radishes, and arugula, provide your body with a potent level of protection against cancer.

It is also important to know that when you eat these veggies, you can gain even more benefit by chewing them really, really well, or blending them in a smoothie, or chopping or dicing them finely. That's because it is necessary to break down the cell walls to activate the anti-cancer compounds.

I am often asked what I eat, and these 100 foods comprise pretty much my whole diet. But it is not enough to know what I have for breakfast, or what I put in my salad at lunch; rather, it is more important to understand why I focus my diet on these 100 particular foods.

These foods comprise the majority of an eating style I term the "Nutritarian Diet." I needed a unique name to emphasize the importance of consuming an adequate amount and variety of micronutrients. The Nutritarian Diet is based on the latest research in the field of nutritional science. The diet is a nutrient-dense, plant-rich (NDPR) eating style that is abundant in vegetables, beans, fresh fruit, nuts, seeds, and intact whole grains.

Some animal products (fish, eggs and dairy) are permitted, but in much smaller quantities than are typically consumed. Eating these healthful, nutrient-dense plant foods will give you the power to take control of your health destiny.

Thousands of scientific studies support the lifespan-promoting effects of eating this kind of nutrient-dense, plant-rich diet. Some of these studies are cited in the following pages for your reference, and many others are on my website: www.drfuhrman.com. When you begin to incorporate this information into your life, the natural effect will be better health, a slimmer waistline, more energy, and protection against illness.

KNOWLEDGE IS POWER

The key to my lifespan-enhancing program is the idea of nutrient density, as shown by this simple formula:

$$H = N / C$$

Health = Nutrients / Calories

This means that your long-term health (H) is determined by the amount of nutrients (N) per calories consumed (C) in your diet throughout life. The goal is to get excellent nutritional intake with fewer calories. Plus, because consuming enough micronutrients prevents overeating behavior, you naturally desire fewer calories.

I hope the information and recipes in this book will encourage you to try foods you've never considered eating before – and to understand more fully why you should strive to eat a varied diet of whole plant foods. If you make these 100 foods the primary focus of what you eat, you'll have the ideal diet.

You won't just live longer—you will live better.

ALMONDS

Almonds have been prized throughout history, and are even mentioned in the Bible's Book of Numbers. Around 100 A.D., Romans showered almonds on newlyweds as a fertility charm.

WHAT MAKES THEM SO SPECIAL?

Eating nuts every day is a good strategy for reducing your risk of heart disease.[1]

Studies on almonds, in particular, have shown that eating them daily increases the amount of antioxidant vitamin E in the blood-stream, improves blood flow, and reduces LDL cholesterol and LDL cholesterol oxidation, along with triglycerides, blood pressure and measures of oxidative stress.[2-6] There have also been studies in healthy people and those with type 2 diabetes showing that adding almonds to the diet improved blood glucose and insulin levels.[4, 7-10]

ALMOND HEMP MILK
SERVES: 6

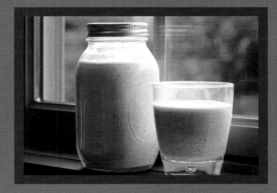

INGREDIENTS

1 cup hulled hemp seeds
1 cup raw almonds, soaked 6-8 hours
2 medjool or 4 regular dates, pitted
4 cups water
1/2 teaspoon vanilla-bean powder

INSTRUCTIONS

1. Place all ingredients in a high pow-ered blender. Blend until smooth.

2. If desired, strain through a nut milk bag or fine mesh strainer.

To make chocolate Nutri Milk, add 2 -3 tablespoons natural cocoa powder to blender along with other ingredients.

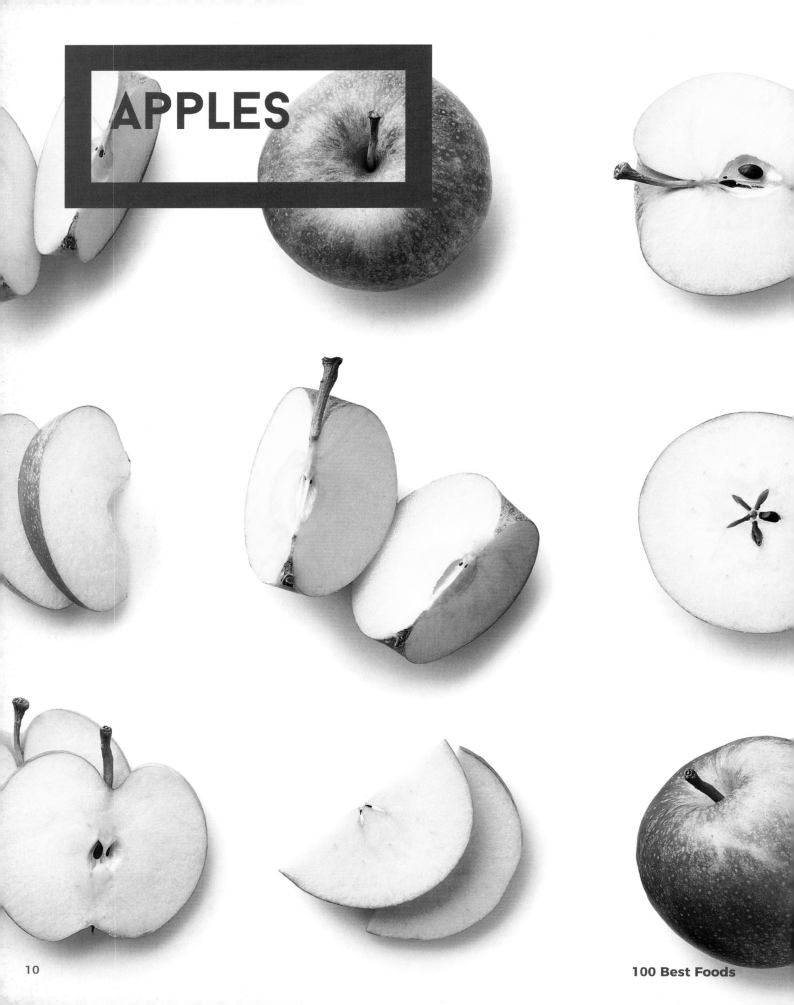

Did you know that the apple is probably the most frequently mentioned fruit in Western art and literature? The Golden Apple was a key element of the Trojan War, and in Norse mythology, magic apples allowed the gods to preserve their immortality. The *Arabian Nights* also features a magic apple – one that can cure any disease. Countless poems feature apples, including those by Robert Frost and Emily Dickinson.

WHAT MAKES THEM SO SPECIAL?

The old adage "an apple a day keeps the doctor away" is continually found to be true. Apple intake has been linked to a lower risk of heart disease.[1] Apple pectin is a soluble fiber, which helps lower cholesterol.[2] Apples also contain polyphenols, which are antioxidants, mostly concentrated in the peel. One of these polyphenols is a flavonoid called epicatechin, which can help lower blood pressure.[1] In a study of over 38,000 women, eating at least one apple a day was linked to a 28 percent lower risk of type 2 diabetes, compared to eating no apples.[3] Observational studies have also linked apples to a lower risk of lung, colorectal, and breast cancers.[4] Purchase organic apples, so you can eat the skin.

DID YOU KNOW...?

A new apple tree produces fruit with characteristics very different from its parent tree, which means that growers can't plant Red Delicious seeds to grow a new Red Delicious tree. They must use a graft of an existing tree to maintain the fruit variety's distinct characteristics.

APPLE PIE OATMEAL
SERVES: 2

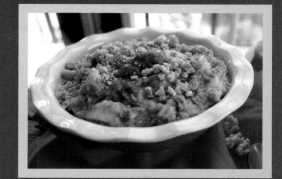

INGREDIENTS
1/2 cup old-fashioned or steel cut oats (see note)
1 cup water
2 apples, peeled, cored, and diced
1/4 teaspoon ground cinnamon
2 regular dates or 1 Medjool date, pitted, finely chopped
2 tablespoons chopped walnuts
1/4 teaspoon vanilla-bean powder

INSTRUCTIONS
1. Place oats and water in small pot and bring to gentle boil. Reduce heat to low and simmer for 5 minutes.

2. Stir in apples, ground cinnamon, and chopped dates. Add additional water if needed to adjust consistency.

3. When oatmeal and apples are heated through, remove from heat and stir in walnuts and vanilla.

Note: If using steel cut oats, double the amount of water and simmer for 20 minutes or until tender.

APRICOTS

Apricots have been prized throughout history for their golden-orange beauty and velvety sweetness. The fruit was first introduced to the New World in the early 18th century by Spanish missionaries in California.

WHAT MAKES THEM SO SPECIAL?

Sure, apricots taste great and have plenty of potassium and soluble fiber to lower cholesterol,[1] but it is their high levels of cancer-defending phytochemicals that make them so special. These phytochemicals include beta-carotene, flavonoids quercetin, catechin, and epicatechin; plus other polyphenols such as caffeic acid, ferulic acid, and cholorogenic acid.[2] Apricots, particularly dried apricots are also a good source of iron. When buying dried apricots make sure they are sulfite-free. Choose fresh fruit that is plump, with a golden or orange-red color; look for fruits with no touch of green whatsoever and give them a sniff – a sweet fragrance indicates that the fruit is flavorful. You can store ripe apricots in the refrigerator for up to a week, but for best flavor and texture, try to use them within two or three days.

DID YOU KNOW...?

In the US, there is something called National Apricot Day. It is observed on 9th of January every year.

ARTICHOKES

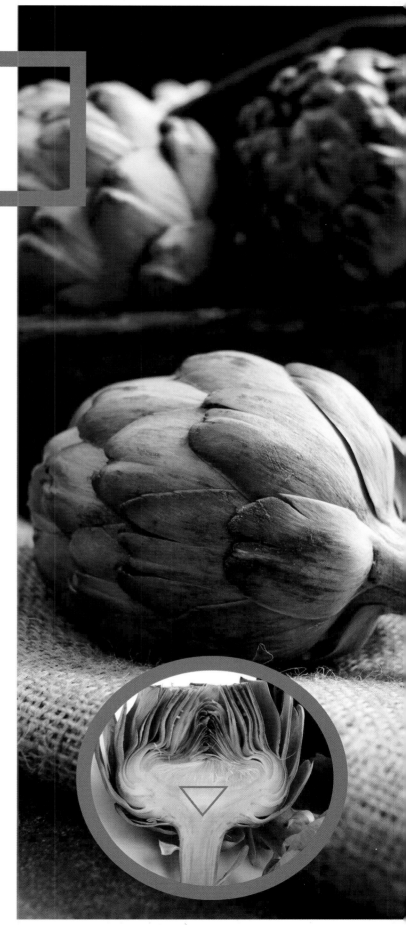

Ancient Greeks and Romans considered artichokes to be a delicacy and an aphrodisiac. In the 16th century, women were not allowed to eat artichokes because of the food's amorous reputation.

WHAT MAKES THEM SO SPECIAL?

Artichokes may seem intimidating, thanks to their armor of thorny leaves, but they are packed with vitamins and minerals, which makes them a valuable addition to a healthy diet. Artichokes are a good source of vitamin K, folate and potassium. One medium artichoke delivers 27 percent of the recommended daily intake of folate. It is also rich in inulin, a prebiotic fiber – meaning that it fuels the growth of beneficial bacteria in the gut.[1, 2]

To prepare, cut about one inch from the top of the artichoke to remove most thorns, and then trim the dark bottom of the stem off, by slicing off about a quarter inch. Cut the artichoke in half and then make a half moon cut with a small sharp knife at the line between the choke and the edible heart, to remove and discard the triangular feathery choke and small inedible leaves right above. Now, the artichoke will steam faster and more evenly, only taking about 18 minutes. Eat the entire heart and stem of the artichoke and all the soft yellow leaves. Scrape off the "meat" under the tough larger leaves with a utensil or your teeth.

ARUGULA

Although arugula goes back to 5th century A.D., it didn't catch on in the U.S. until it started to become trendy in the 1980s. In ancient Greece and Rome, consumption of arugula was associated with aphrodisiac properties.

WHAT MAKES IT SO SPECIAL?

Arugula is a cruciferous vegetable. Among other things, the phytochemicals in cruciferous vegetables activate protective biochemical pathways in our cells, which help to promote cardiovascular health and reduce the risk of cancer. Arugula is also high in vital nutrients, like vitamin K, which maintains strong bones. Erucin, an isothiocyanate (ITC) derived specifically from arugula, has been shown to slow growth of cancerous cells in vitro and also to have anti-inflammatory effects.[1, 2] A research group also determined that an arugula extract may even help to treat gastric ulcers.[3] The greatest thing about arugula compared to other cruciferous vegetables is that it is eaten raw in salads, rather than cooked, leaving its enzymes fully intact.

In addition to adding a peppery flavor to salads, this versatile green can be added to soups. Add a few handfuls of arugula just after your soup has finished cooking – the tender green leaves will wilt very quickly. Or toss arugula into a pasta dish while adding sauce. Top each serving with a handful of raw arugula to increase the ITC content.

DID YOU KNOW...?

Arugula is also known by other names such as rocket, roquette, rucola, rugula.

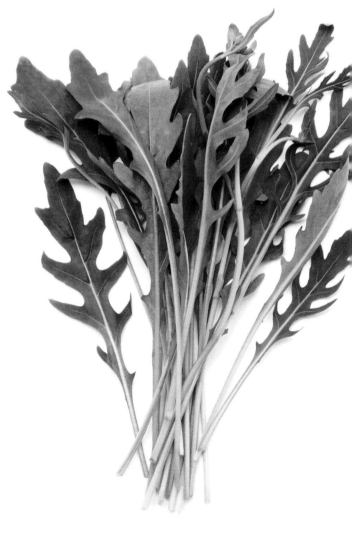

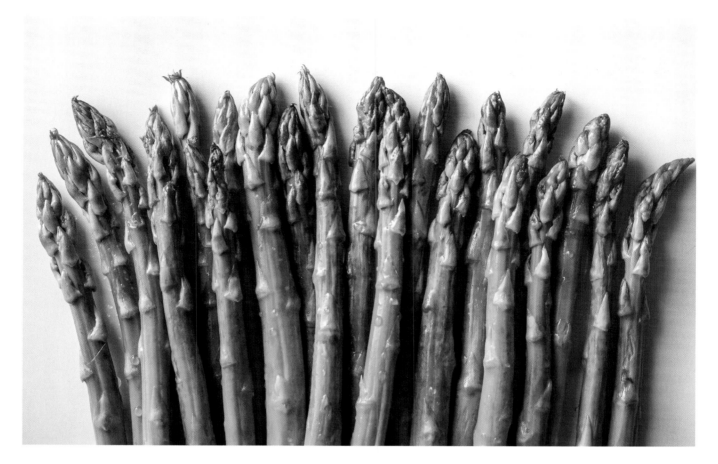

ASPARAGUS

Asparagus has been hailed as a miracle vegetable since ancient times. The Greeks believed asparagus could cure a number of ailments, from toothaches to heart disease.

WHAT MAKES IT SO SPECIAL?

Asparagus provides more folate than almost any other vegetable (only raw spinach and turnip greens have more). In addition to its importance in fetal brain development, folate is essential throughout life. Natural folate, a B vitamin acquired from food, helps protect against cancer,[1, 2] whereas excess from the synthetic form of folate – folic acid – may be cancer-promoting.[2-4] Asparagus also contains the antioxidants rutin and glutathione, and the flavonol quercetin, which help to keep blood pressure down.[5-7]

DID YOU KNOW...?

It is easy to plant asparagus in your garden, because you don't have to replant it year after year; you just pick it and eat it every year without any additional work involved. Once picked, asparagus loses its flavor and tenderness over time, so enjoy it within a day or two.

AVO TOAST
SERVES: 1

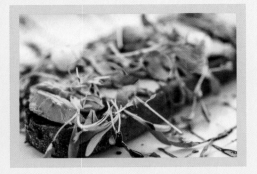

INGREDIENTS

2 (100% whole grain) slices of toast
1/2 ripe avocado, mashed
1/2 tomato, sliced
handful of arugula
drizzle of balsamic vinegar
black pepper or red pepper flakes,
to taste

INSTRUCTIONS

1. Spread the mashed avocado on top of toast.

2. Add tomato slices.

3. Top with arugula and drizzle with balsamic vinegar.

4. Season with your choice of ground black pepper or red pepper flakes.

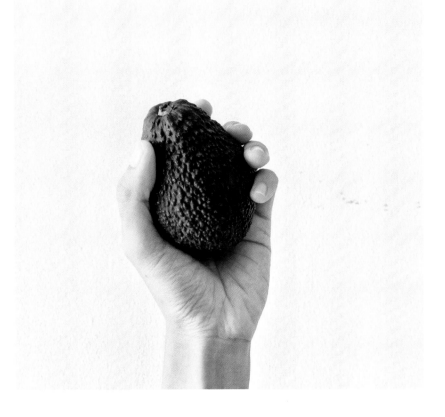

AVOCADO

Avocados (also called alligator pears) are the fruit with the highest amount of fat and protein. A Hass avocado usually contains about 4 grams of protein and a whopping 10 grams of fiber. In order to harvest avocados, workers use a long pole to snip fruit from the tree, and catch it in a mesh or canvas bag. They can ripen on or off the tree.

WHAT MAKES IT SO SPECIAL?

Eating avocados may lower your risk for heart disease, diabetes and stroke.[1] Several studies show that eating avocados may offer benefits such as decreased total cholesterol, LDL cholesterol and triglycerides. [2] Promoting healthy blood lipid profiles is not the only reason to eat them: adding half an avocado to lunch has been shown to increase meal satisfaction, and reduce the desire to eat more over the next few hours.[3] Also, when eaten with other fruits and vegetables, the fat content of avocados helps to enhance the bioavailability of the fat-soluble nutrients from these other foods.[4]

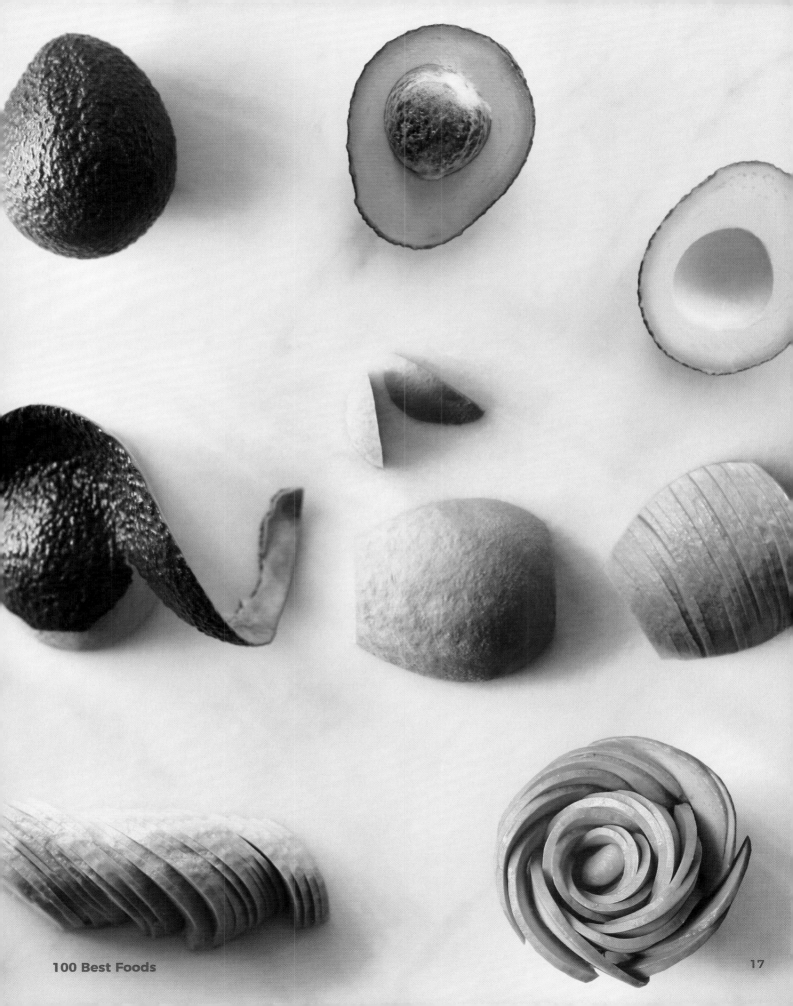

BANANAS

Bananas, which are grown in tropical climates, are picked green. Upon arrival in the destination country, they are placed in rooms filled with ethylene gas to induce ripening. The vivid yellow color you see in supermarkets is actually caused by this artificial ripening process.

WHAT MAKES THEM SO SPECIAL?

Although not as colorful and rich in antioxidants as fruits such as cherries, pomegranate or berries, bananas still contain significant antioxidants, primarily phenolic compounds.

They also contain a good amount of fiber, pectin, fructooligosaccharides, and resistant starch (the less ripe the banana, the more resistant starch). All these components fuel the growth of beneficial gut bacteria, resulting in a number of health benefits, including protecting against colon cancer.[1,2] Bananas also provide potassium and other electrolyte minerals, B vitamins, selenium and carotenoids. Bananas are Americans' favorite fruit – 18 million tons were consumed in 2015 alone. Plantains are a type of large banana that is often cooked like a starchy vegetable, before it is fully ripe, but can be allowed to ripen and eaten raw. Interestingly the skin of the banana can be eaten raw or cooked (only if organic), but does not taste very good; that's why even monkeys discard it.

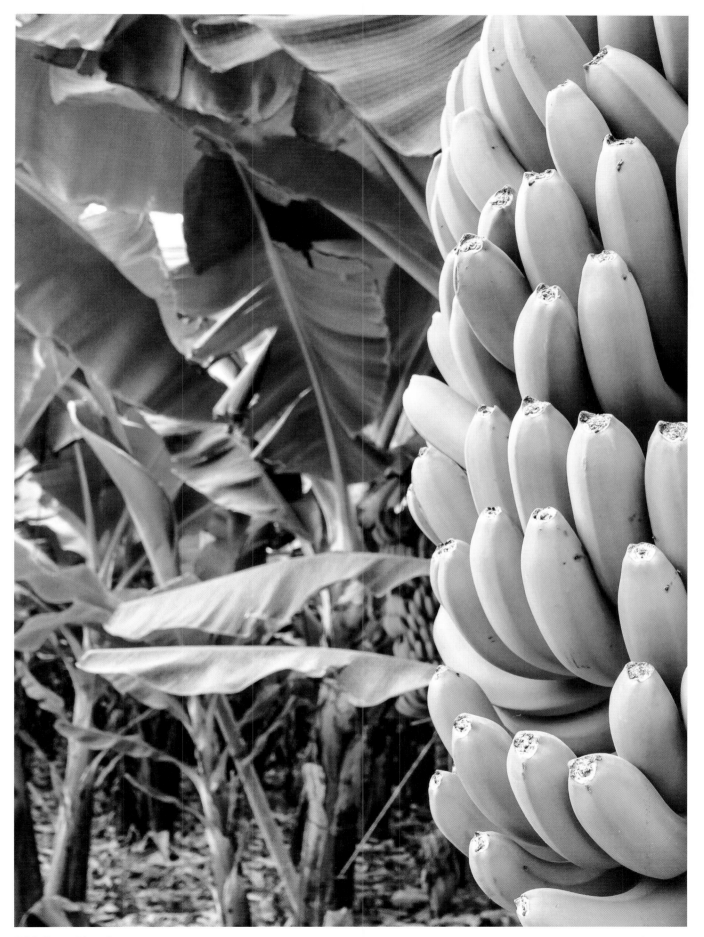

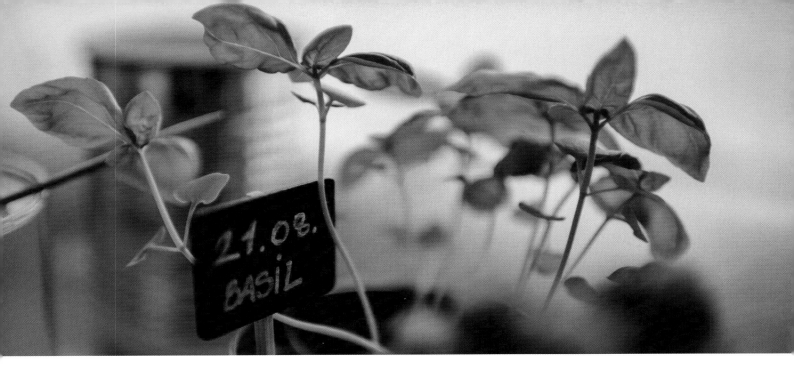

BASIL

In ancient Egypt, basil is thought to have been one of the fragrant herbs used as an embalming ingredient, to prepare bodies for mummification. There are many varieties of basil, including the sweet basil used in Italian cooking, Thai basil, and tulsi or holy basil, which is considered sacred in the Hindu religion.

WHAT MAKES IT SO SPECIAL?

Basil is a high-antioxidant food,[1] and purple basil has higher free radical scavenging power than green because of the presence of anthocyanins – the same flavonoid phytochemicals that give berries their deep blue, red, and purple colors.[2] Studies on human white blood cells showed that components of sweet basil were found to have strong anti-inflammatory activity.[3] Another notable feature of basil is its ability to impede the growth of microorganisms.[2] Basil extracts in laboratory studies showed effectiveness at inhibiting the growth of a number of strains of harmful bacteria.[4-6]

DID YOU KNOW...?

Linalool, a phytochemical found in basil, naturally repels mosquitoes.[7]

LEMON BASIL VINAIGRETTE
SERVES: 4

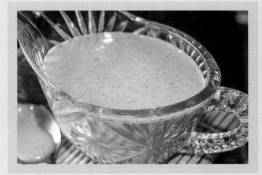

INGREDIENTS
2 tablespoons fresh lemon juice
2 tablespoons balsamic vinegar
1/2 cup water
1/4 cup raw almonds
1/4 cup raisins
1/3 cup fresh basil leaves
1 teaspoon Dijon mustard
1 clove garlic

INSTRUCTIONS
1. Blend ingredients in a high-powered blender until smooth.

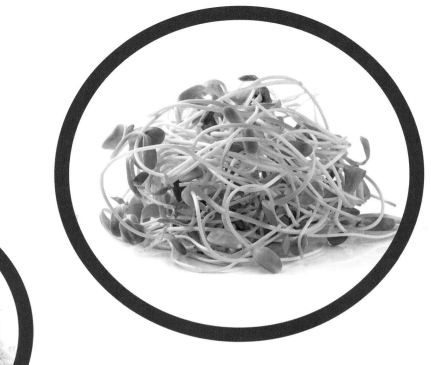

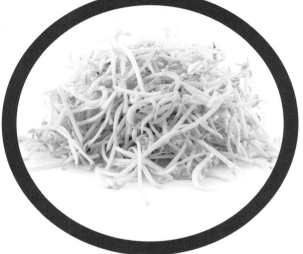

BEAN SPROUTS

Sprouts have long been used for food as well as for medicine. Over 5,000 years ago, Chinese physicians prescribed sprouts for curing many disorders. Sprouts are a staple ingredient in Asian cuisine in the U.S. and in Asian countries. However, it took centuries for the West to fully realize the food's nutritional merits.

WHAT MAKES THEM SO SPECIAL?
The sprouted seeds of legumes such as lentils, soy beans, or mung beans have a somewhat different nutritional profile than the seeds do in their unsprouted form. Sprouted seeds are richer in calcium, vitamin C and antioxidant compounds than their unsprouted counterparts, and the protein is often more digestible.[1-3] Studies on mung bean sprouts have revealed their toxic effects on cancer cells.[4]

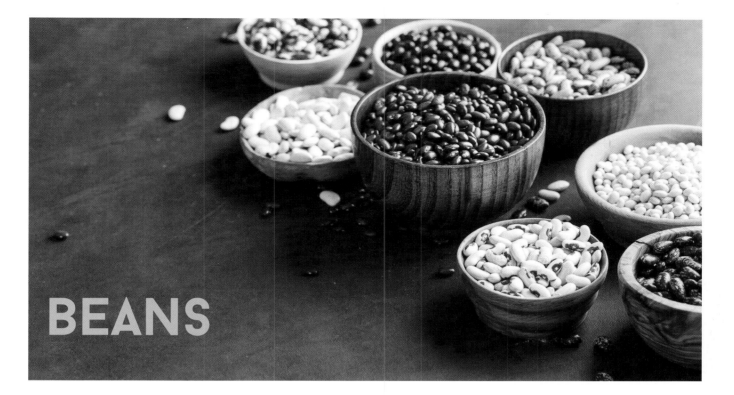

BEANS

Beans are a heliotropic plant, meaning that the leaves tilt throughout the day to face the sun. At night, they go into a folded "sleep" position. Beans come in an array of colors, shapes and sizes, with over 4,000 varieties. This huge diversity is the result of the very nature of the bean itself. Its constant transformation from generation to generation results in new combinations of color, and a vast array of other genetic features.

WHAT MAKES THEM SO SPECIAL?

In my book *Super Immunity*, I explain how a diet with a portfolio of immune system-strengthening and cancer-fighting foods creates enhanced protection for your health. Beans make up a vital part of this health-supporting diet style. Since they are high-nutrient, high-fiber, low-calorie foods, beans are effective as a weight loss tool. They are also the ideal starch source – high-nutrient and low-glycemic – for people with diabetes or prediabetes. Beans provide plenty of protein, fiber, folate, iron, potassium and magnesium, along with just a moderate amount of calories. People who eat beans regularly have greater intakes of minerals and fiber, have lower blood pressure, and are less likely to be overweight than those who don't.[1] Randomized controlled trials that added legumes to participants' diets have reported reduced blood pressure, cholesterol, fasting blood glucose, and C-reactive protein levels (which is a measure of inflamation).[2-5] Many studies have shown that greater consumption of beans is associated with a lower risk of colorectal cancer and prostate cancer.[6,7] Besides their high amount of resistant starch and fiber, which fuel the growth of favorable bacteria in the gut, they also contain lots of polyphenols and other anti-cancer phytochemicals, which explains the powerful protection they offer against cancers, especially breast cancer.[8-11]

DID YOU KNOW...?

Canned beans are a convenient option, but beans in boxes are also a great choice. Look for "no-salt-added" beans, and don't waste the liquid they come with – it is rich in nutrients, and can be used in soups and stews.

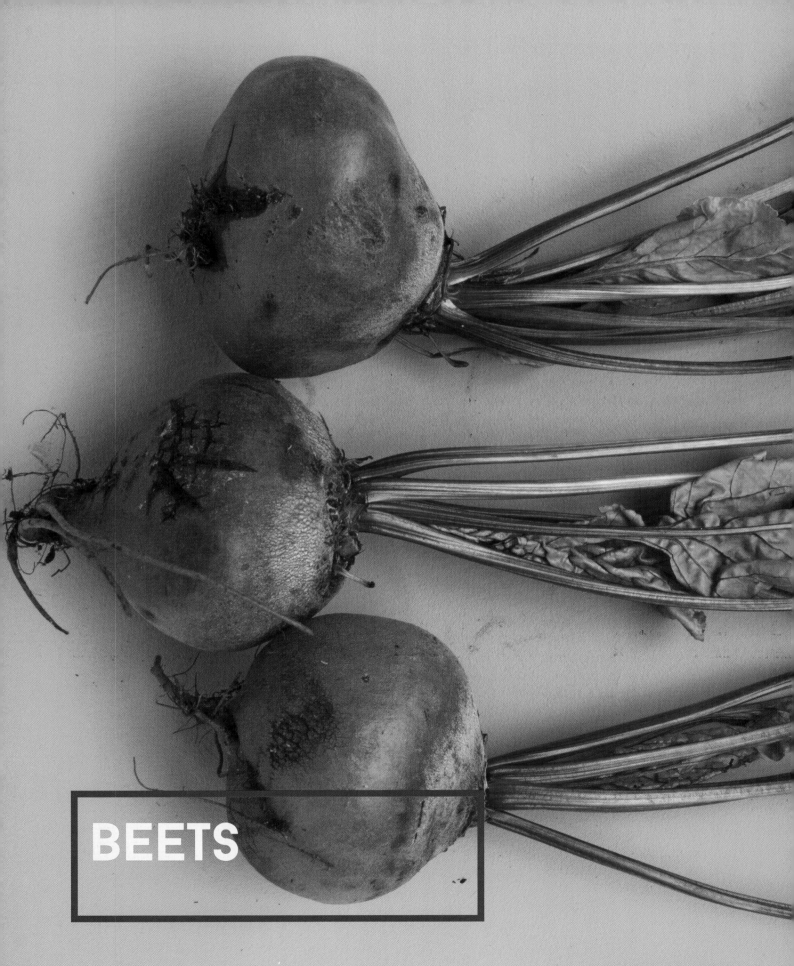

BEETS

Beet or beetroot, as it is commonly called outside the United States, was domesticated in the Middle East in the 8th century B.C. Betanin, obtained from the roots of a beet, is used industrially as a natural red food colorant as well as a colorant in cosmetics and pharmaceuticals.

WHAT MAKES THEM SO SPECIAL?

The high nitrate content of beets increases blood nitric oxide concentrations, which may help prevent heart disease by lowering blood pressure. In addition, the nitric oxide in beet juice has been linked to improved endurance in high-intensity exercise performance in several studies.[1,2] In one study, subjects given two-thirds of a cup of concentrated beet juice saw an immediate increase of 13 percent in their muscle capacity. Aside from the nitric oxide, beets also contain unique health-boosting nutrients that you may not be getting elsewhere. They are an exceptional source of betalains, a group of phytochemicals (including betacyanins and betaxanthins) that protect cells against oxidative damage and inflammation.[3] In addition, the betalain pigments in beets support the body's phase II detoxification process, which is when broken-down toxins are bound to other molecules so they can be excreted from your body.[3]

DID YOU KNOW...?

The green leaves of beets are edible and packed with carotenoids, minerals, protein and fiber – just one cup provides 17 percent of your daily fiber requirement. Add them to your salads for a nutritional boost.

BEET HUMMUS
SERVES: 4

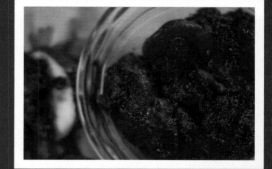

INGREDIENTS

3 medium beets, scrubbed
2 large garlic cloves
1 (15 ounce) can no-salt-added or low-sodium chick peas, drained
1/4 cup unhulled sesame seeds, lightly toasted
2 tablespoons water
2 tablespoons lemon juice
1 teaspoon ground cumin
pinch black pepper

INSTRUCTIONS

1. Preheat oven to 375 degrees F.

2. Place beets and garlic cloves on a sheet of foil. Fold up and bake for 45 minutes or until beets are tender when pierced with a knife.

3. Remove skins from garlic and beets.

4. Place beets, garlic, chick peas, sesame seeds, water, lemon juice, cumin and black pepper in a food processor or high-powered blender and pulse until smooth.

5. Serve on top of sliced cucumber or zucchini rounds or as a dip with assorted raw vegetables.

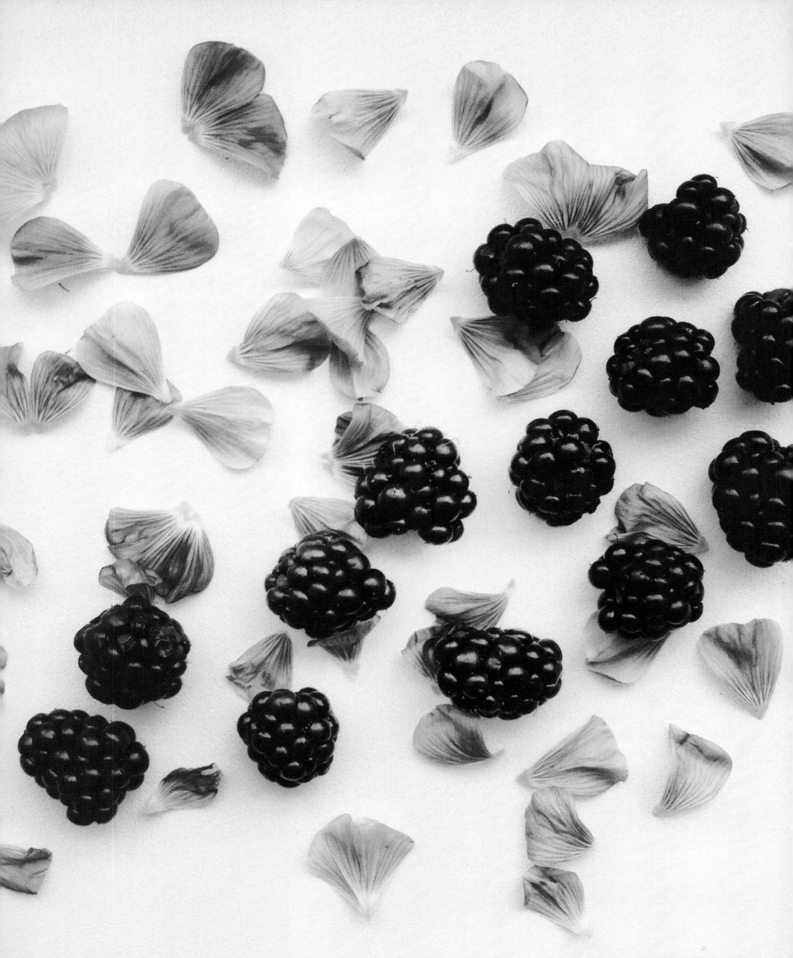

BLACKBERRIES

The blackberry plant has been used to treat ailments ranging from diarrhea to scurvy dating all the way back to ancient Greece. The very dark color of blackberries is evidence of the high antioxidant levels contained in the fruit.

WHAT MAKES THEM SO SPECIAL?

Blackberry fruit contains phytochemicals that have strong anti-cancer effects; they prevent DNA damage and the proliferation of cancer cells in vitro and in animals. Blackberries' anti-cancer effects have been attributed to the abundance of anthocyanins – responsible for the deep purple to black color of the berries – and other phytochemicals, such as ellagic acid.[1] Blackberries are also valuable for keeping inflammation in check, which has been demonstrated in humans. In a randomized controlled trial in which 72 patients supplemented with pulp-containing blackberry juice or followed their usual diet for eight weeks, C-reactive protein (a marker of inflammation) decreased in the blackberry group compared to control group.[2] These berries, with their potent dark anthocyanins, should be consumed often for many reasons.

DID YOU KNOW...?

Blackberries can be found growing in the wild and are also known as Brambleberries, so named for the Bramble, the thorny bush on which they grow.

BLUEBERRIES

Although largely associated with Maine, the world can thank New Jersey – and, specifically, a woman named Elizabeth White – for domesticating and commercializing the berry in the early 20th century. In 1911, White teamed up with USDA botanist Frederick Coville to identify wild plants with the largest berries and most desirable properties. After crossbreeding the bushes, White and Colville grew the new varieties of blueberries in the acidic soil of the Pine Barrens, where they flourished. In 1916, the pair harvested and sold the first commercial crop of blueberries.

WHAT MAKES THEM SO SPECIAL?

Blueberry supplementation in several studies improved glucose metabolism in patients with type 2 diabetes.[1] Berry flavonoids are thought to improve nitric oxide availability in the blood vessels, supporting the ability of the arteries to dilate.[2] Compared to eating no blueberries, just one serving per week was associated with a 10 percent decreased risk of hypertension.[3, 4] Blueberries also improve brain health. Studies in older adults have found that those with mild memory problems who supplemented with blueberry juice improved their performance on tests of cognitive function compared to the control groups.[5, 6] Berry flavonoids plus another berry phytochemical, ellagic acid, also have anti-cancer properties: scavenging free radicals, preventing DNA damage, promoting DNA repair, and counteracting inflammation and cancer cell proliferation.[7, 8]

BLUEBERRY CHIA SOAKED OATS
SERVES: 1

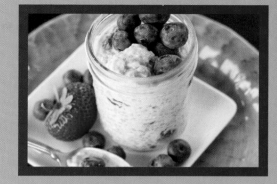

INGREDIENTS

1/2 cup old-fashioned oats
1 tablespoon chia seeds
1 cup unsweetened soy, hemp or almond milk
2 tablespoons raisins
1/2 cup fresh or thawed frozen blueberries (or other fruit)

INSTRUCTIONS

1. Combine the oats, chia seeds, non-dairy milk and raisins.

2. Soak for at least 30 minutes or overnight.

3. Stir in blueberries.

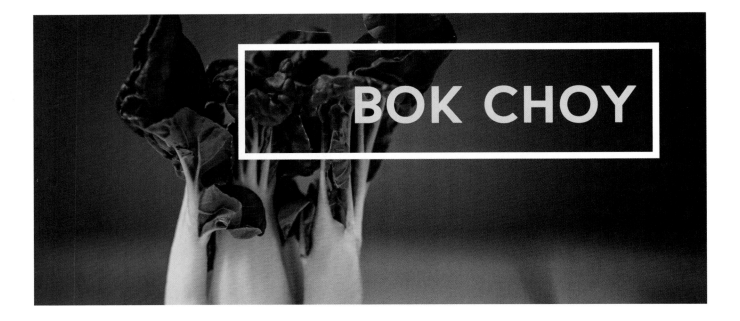

BOK CHOY

Although less familiar in American cuisine, the Chinese have been cultivating bok choy, also called pak choi, for more than 5,000 years.

WHAT MAKES IT SO SPECIAL?

Improved heart health, bone health, cancer protection, and immune health are among the potential benefits of eating bok choy regularly.

This vegetable is so high in beta-carotene (which the body converts to vitamin A), that just one cup of cooked bok choy provides enough vitamin A to exceed the daily recommended intake.[1] Beta-carotene and other carotenoids found in bok choy scavenge free radicals, and vitamin A is essential for the health of the retina and other parts of the eye.

For this reason, foods high in carotenoids may help those who are suffering from – or at risk for – Age-related Macular Degeneration, a disease of the eyes that is a common cause of vision loss in older adults.[1]

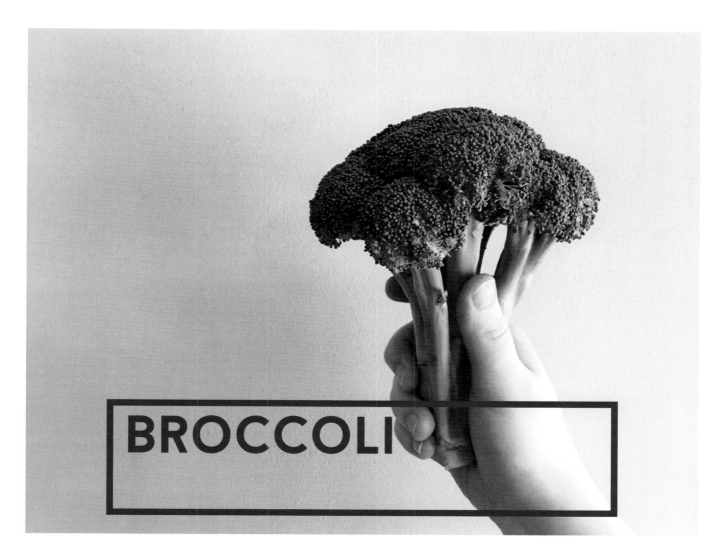

BROCCOLI

Ciao bella, broccoli! This cruciferous vegetable, a relative of cabbage, was cultivated in Italy as far back as ancient Rome, and came to the Americas and England in the 1700s. Great for the waistline, broccoli is high in protein and fiber, yet very low in calories, at only 30 calories per cup.

WHAT MAKES IT SO SPECIAL?

Broccoli's powerful combination of antioxidant, anti-inflammatory and detoxification properties makes it an extraordinary food in cancer prevention.
Isothiocyanates (ITCs) in cruciferous vegetables have many different cancer-fighting effects. Studies have suggested that sulforaphane – an ITC present in high concentrations in broccoli – enhances antioxidant protection, accelerates the detoxification of carcinogens, inhibits the growth and proliferation of cancerous cells, and helps reduce inflammation in the cardiovascular system.[1]

> Broccoli is a great food to grow in your garden or in a grow box. Broccoli florets are the flower of the plant, but the leaves are edible and even more nutritious. Pull the leaves off the plant while it is growing and get the plant's full benefit.

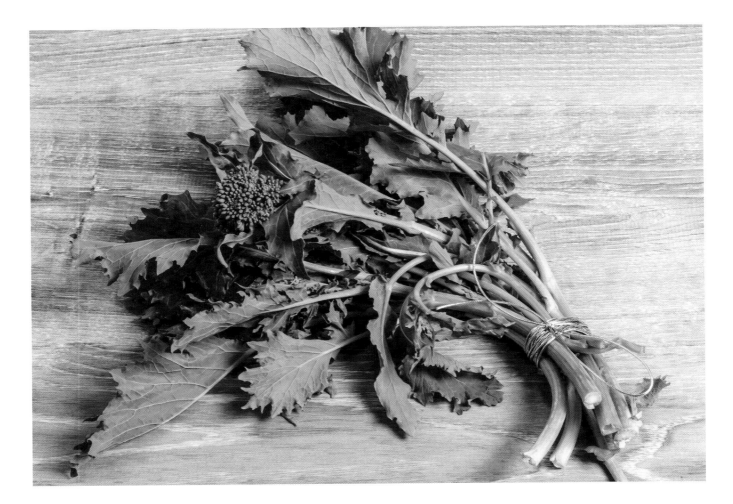

BROCCOLI RABE

Despite its name, this cruciferous green vegetable is more similar to mustard greens or turnip greens than it is to broccoli, especially in regard to taste. Its bitter, nutty flavor mellows when cooked, but it still remains pungent.

WHAT MAKES IT SO SPECIAL?

Broccoli rabe's mild bitterness reflects the potent amount of isothiocyanates it contains. That's why this cruciferous vegetable is such a powerful anti-cancer food.[1-3] Just one cup of broccoli rabe meets the recommended vitamin K intake for the day.

DID YOU KNOW...?

If you find broccoli rabe's bitterness overwhelming, blanch it for one minute in boiling water, then drain and season to taste.

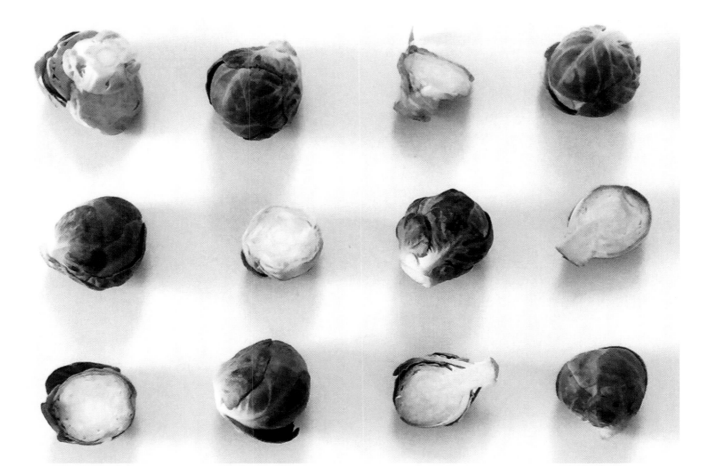

BRUSSELS SPROUTS

While Brussels sprouts were named after the capital city of Belgium, it is believed that a forerunner of this tiny green vegetable was grown in ancient Rome as well.

Have you ever wondered why some people strongly dislike the taste of Brussels sprouts while others love them? Those in the "dislike" camp aren't being overly picky – their distaste for this particular taste is caused by a pattern of variants in the taste receptor gene TAS2R38, which allows them to detect certain bitter flavor compounds in Brussels sprouts and additional cruciferous vegetables, coffee and other bitter foods. People with the "non-tasting" variants tend to detect less bitterness in these foods, and may enjoy them more as a result.[1] Hopefully, you love Brussels sprouts, because this cruciferous vegetable is high on the list of superfoods.

WHAT MAKES THEM SO SPECIAL?

This classic fall vegetable is a nutritional powerhouse, with many health benefits. As with other cruciferous relatives, the phytochemicals in Brussels sprouts have been identified as having cancer-preventive effects. For example, Brussels sprouts may protect DNA from damage due to carcinogens and oxidants. A study of people who consumed about 10 ounces of Brussels sprouts daily showed improved stability of DNA in their white blood cells.[2]

CABBAGE
NAPA AND RED

Cabbage is part of the cruciferous family of vegetables. **Red cabbage** comes in various shades of dark red/purple according to the pH of the soil. In acidic conditions, the color is red, in neutral soil it's purple, and in alkaline conditions, it's blue-green. **Napa cabbage** (a type of Chinese cabbage) is sweeter and milder than its standard green cousin; historians believe it is a naturally hybridized cross between bok choy and a turnip.

NAPA (CHINESE) CABBAGE

WHAT MAKES IT SO SPECIAL?

Napa cabbage, like all green vegetables, is high in folate, and like other cruciferous vegetables is a source of isothiocyanates (ITCs), which contribute their powerful anti-cancer benefits.[1] We get the biggest ITC boost if we eat our cruciferous vegetables raw and chew them well. Napa cabbage provides an excellent way to eat raw cruciferous, because it's delicious when sliced thinly and added to salads and slaws.

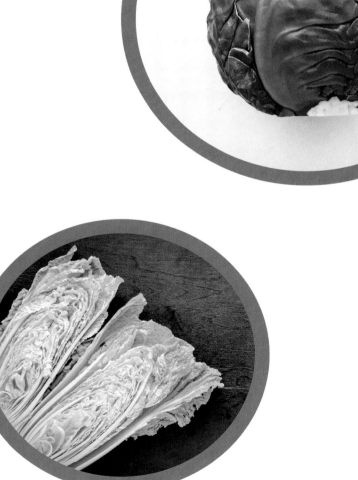

RED CABBAGE

WHAT MAKES IT SO SPECIAL?

Red cabbage outshines its standard green cousin when it comes to nutritional value. Red cabbage has the phytochemicals found in all cruciferous vegetables, plus anthocyanins (the cardioprotective and anti-inflammatory phytochemicals characteristic of berries) which provide the red/purple color. Cruciferous phytochemicals have properties that help to suppress some of the processes vital to the development of cancer, such as cell proliferation, angiogenesis, and metastasis. Having just a few servings per week of cruciferous vegetables has been linked to protection from several types of cancer, including prostate, lung, breast, colon, ovarian, and bladder cancers.[2-7]

DID YOU KNOW...?

Testing pH with red cabbage juice is a popular kids' science experiment, since the anthocyanins change color depending on how acidic or alkaline the solution is.

NAPA CABBAGE AND KALE SLAW
SERVES: 4

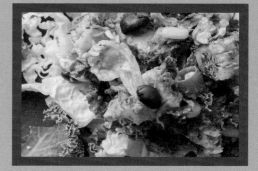

INGREDIENTS
SALAD
2 cups kale, finely chopped
2 heads Napa cabbage, finely chopped
3 green onions, chopped
1 cup cooked beans, any variety
1 cup fresh or defrosted frozen corn kernels
1 ripe avocado, cubed
1/4 cup fresh parsley

DRESSING
3 tablespoons unsalted peanut butter
6 tablespoons warm water
1 medjool or 2 regular dates, pitted and mashed
1 tablespoon apple cider vinegar
1 teaspoon reduced-sodium miso
1/4 teaspoon grated ginger
1/4 teaspoon lemon grass paste, optional

INSTRUCTIONS
1. Place the salad ingredients in a large bowl and combine.

2. Whisk or use a blender to blend the peanut butter, water, date, vinegar, miso, ginger and lemon grass paste. Toss with dressing. Refrigerate at least one hour and toss again before serving.

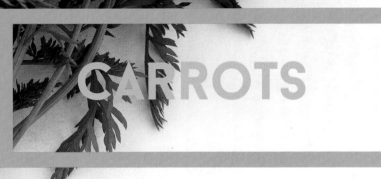

CARROTS

We tend to think of carrots as being bright orange, but they actually come in a range of colors, including white, purple, yellow, and red. The debate is still on as to how carrots became ubiquitously orange: one (unconfirmed) theory is that 17th century Dutch farmers cultivated the vegetable in this color to honor their monarch, William of Orange.

WHAT MAKES THEM SO SPECIAL?

Carrots are powerhouses of the immune-boosting carotenoids beta-carotene, alpha-carotene and beta-cryptoxanthin, all of which are antioxidants and convert to vitamin A in the body. Vitamin A is essential for the maintenance of good vision, sperm production, skin integrity, and normal growth and development; high blood carotenoid levels are linked to longevity.[1-3] There is also evidence that the carrot phytochemical falcarinol may help to prevent colon cancer.[4]

Eating raw vegetables, such as carrots and broccoli, helps make for comfortable bowel movements. However, eating cooked carrots may be better for absorption of carotenoids, which become more bioavailable once vegetables have been heated.[5] A University of Arkansas study found that cooked, pureed carrots had a higher antioxidant capacity than their raw counterparts.[6] So eat them both raw and cooked. Enjoy raw carrots or other carotenoid-rich foods with a nut-based dip or dressing. The fat from the nuts increases carotenoid absorption from the carrots.[7]

100 Best Foods

CASHEWS

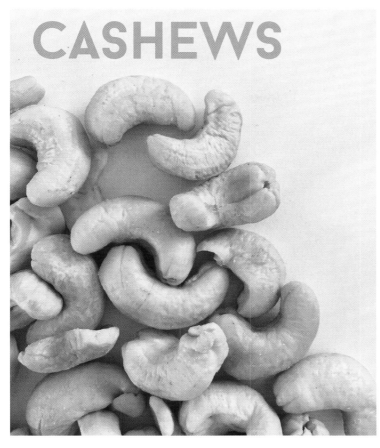

Ever wonder why you never see cashew nuts for sale in their shells? It's because the double shells surrounding cashews contain a potent skin irritant that is chemically related to the allergenic oil found in poison ivy. The cashew shell grows at the end of the sweet-flavored cashew apple, which is often used in India to make jams and chutneys.

WHAT MAKES THEM SO SPECIAL?

Cashews are rich in minerals, providing significant amounts of magnesium, iron, zinc, copper, and manganese. Overall, daily consumption of nuts is linked to a lower risk of heart disease, maintaining a healthy weight, and living longer.[1-4] In a study on patients with type 2 diabetes, adding about one ounce of cashews to the diet for 12 weeks reduced systolic blood pressure compared to the control group.[5] A similar, one-month-long study found a reduction in total and LDL cholesterol levels.[6]

DID YOU KNOW…?

There is no such thing as eating a truly raw cashew. Due to their outer layers being toxic, they go through the following processes before being sold: dried, steamed, shelled, peeled, graded and roasted at low heat.

TOFU CASHEW REMOULADE
SERVES: 10

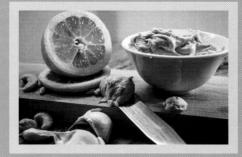

INGREDIENTS

12 ounces silken tofu, like Mori-Nu brand
1/2 cup raw cashews, soaked in water to cover for 15-30 minutes
2 tablespoons lemon juice
1 teaspoon Braggs Liquid Aminos
2 tablespoons rice vinegar
1 tablespoon whole grain mustard
2-3 tablespoons tomato paste, to adjust color to a light red
1 teaspoon paprika, or more to taste
1 teaspoon grated horseradish root, or more to taste
1-2 teaspoons chipotle or ancho chile powder, to taste

INSTRUCTIONS

1. Add tofu, cashews with the soaking water and the remaining ingredients to a high-powered blender and blend until smooth.

2. Add more water if necessary to adjust consistency. Taste for desired heat and adjust if required, best to start with smaller amounts and add more after tasting.

Use as a salad dressing, dip or burger topping.

BUFFALO CAULIFLOWER

SERVES: 4

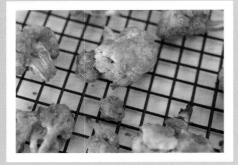

INGREDIENTS

1 cup almond flour
1/4 cup nutritional yeast
1 teaspoon Dr. Fuhrman's MatoZest
or other no-salt seasoning blend,
adjusted to taste
1 teaspoon paprika
1/4-1/2 teaspoon cayenne pepper,
or to taste
2/3 cup water
1 tablespoon Dijon mustard
1 head cauliflower, cut into florets

INSTRUCTIONS

1. Preheat oven to 350° F.

2. Combine flour, nutritional yeast
and seasonings in a bowl.

3. Using a whisk, add water gradually. Stir in mustard. Mixture should
resemble a thick batter.

4. Toss cauliflower florets with the
coating. Place on a parchment-lined
baking sheet and bake for 20-25
minutes until coating is dry and
cauliflower is tender.

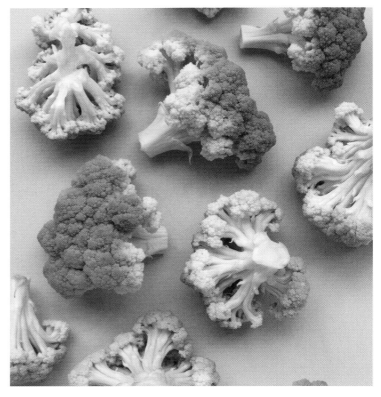

CAULIFLOWER

Cauliflower originally came from Cyprus and was
introduced to France from Italy in the middle of the
16th century. It was all the rage at the court of French
king Louis XIV, where it was served in rich and elegant
dishes. Today, cauliflower has gained considerable
popularity as a low-calorie, low-glycemic alternative to
rice, mashed potatoes and traditional pizza crust.

WHAT MAKES IT SO SPECIAL?

Cauliflower is part of the cruciferous family, and
its glucosinolates, sinigrin and glucobrassicin, are
converted to compounds known to inhibit the growth
of cultured cancer cells.[1] These compounds are likely the
reason for the link between cruciferous vegetable intake
and a reduced risk of common cancers. [2-7] In addition,
cauliflower is a good source of choline, a B vitamin
that is important during pregnancy for its role in brain
development. Higher choline intake during pregnancy
has been associated with a lower risk of neural tube
defects and better visual memory in children at age 7.[8-10]

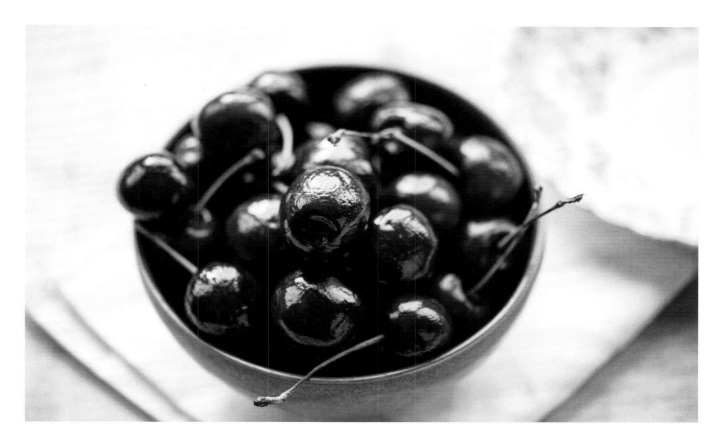

CHERRIES

Although some varieties of cherries are native to North America, the type we are most familiar with came to the United States on the ships of settlers in the 17th century. Cherries are known to have a very short fruiting season, only bearing fruit from late spring to early summer.

WHAT MAKES THEM SO SPECIAL?

Sore post-workout? Tart cherries may help. Studies on cherry supplementation coupled with exercise have shown that those eating cherries had reduced muscle soreness and lesser signs of muscle damage compared to placebo groups, likely because of the anti-inflammatory effects of cherry phytochemicals.[1-4] Cherries also offer cardiovascular benefits, such as lowering C-reactive protein and blood pressure levels.[5-7] Cherry consumption reduces circulating levels of uric acid, which may help patients with gout.[8] Both sweet and sour cherries protect against oxidative stress and inflammation with their rich supply of phytochemicals, including phenolic acids, quercetin and kaempferol;[9, 10] and tart cherries may also improve your sleep, as it is one of the few rich food sources of the hormone melatonin, which regulates our sleep-wake cycle.[11,12]

DID YOU KNOW...?

I cannot tell a lie – the story of George Washington and the cherry tree is actually a myth invented by one of Washington's early biographers! Rev. Mason Locke Weems included it in the fifth edition of his 1800 book, *The Life of Washington,* to present his subject as a model of virtue to inspire children.

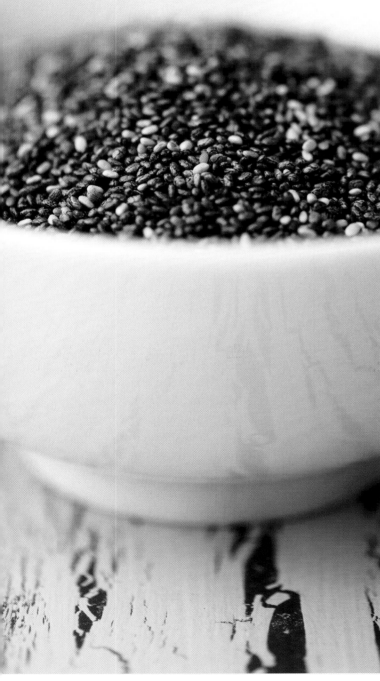

CHIA SEEDS

Although they have been a dietary staple for thousands of years, it's only in the last decade or so that chia seeds have become recognized as a superfood. Chia seeds were an important food for the Aztecs and Mayans, who prized them for their ability to provide sustainable energy.

WHAT MAKES THEM SO SPECIAL?

Don't be misled by size. These tiny seeds are weighty in nutritional benefits, and they are packed – about 18 percent by weight – with the omega-3 fatty acid ALA.[1] In addition to ALA, chia seeds are a good source of fiber (soluble fiber in particular), calcium and magnesium. Human studies in which subjects supplemented with chia seeds daily found that indicators of inflammation and oxidative stress dropped, and so did blood pressure in patients with type 2 diabetes or hypertension.[2-4] Chia seeds are one of the richest sources of lignans, linked to powerful protection from breast and prostate cancer.[5-7]

DID YOU KNOW...?

Because chia seeds absorb so much water and form a gel when placed in liquid, making chia pudding is an easy and delicious way to eat these seeds. Actually, the mild flavor and compact size is such that you can add a spoonful into pretty much anything – so test it, and enjoy its super health benefits. Storing chia seeds in a glass jar in the refrigerator will extend their shelf life.

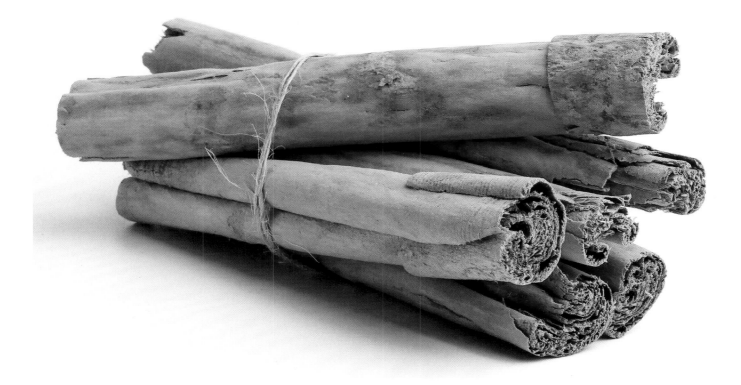

CINNAMON

The high demand for cinnamon kept European explorers busy during the 15th and 16th centuries, and led to a couple of wars. In 1518, the Portuguese seized the island of Ceylon (now Sri Lanka), and controlled the cinnamon trade in Europe. In 1638 they were ousted by the Dutch, who, in turn, were defeated by the British in the Anglo-Dutch war in 1784. Today, most Ceylon cinnamon is still grown in Sri Lanka.

WHAT MAKES IT SO SPECIAL?

This super spice, from the bark of Cinnamomum trees, is chock-full of protective antioxidants that reduce free radical damage and help slow the aging process. But all store-bought cinnamon is not equal. The two main varieties are Ceylon cinnamon (known as "true cinnamon"), and the cheaper, more widely-available Cassia cinnamon. Cassia contains coumarin, a naturally occurring substance that has the potential to damage the liver in high doses.[1, 2] In contrast, Ceylon contains only insignificant traces of coumarin; therefore, it is a better choice if using regularly and liberally.[3]

Anti-inflammatory effects of Ceylon and Cassia cinnamon have been observed, due in large part due to cinnamaldehyde, which also provides cinnamon with much of its flavor.[4, 5] The most interesting property of cinnamon is the ability of its phytochemicals to lower blood sugar.[6]

CHOCOLATE NICE CREAM
SERVES: 2

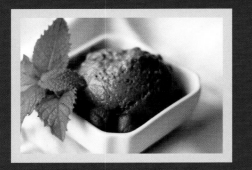

INGREDIENTS

2 large bananas, frozen (see note)
1 teaspoon alcohol-free vanilla extract or vanilla bean powder
2 tablespoons unsweetened soy, hemp or almond milk
2 regular dates or 1 medjool date, pitted
1-2 tablespoons unsweetened cocoa powder

INSTRUCTIONS

1. Place non-dairy milk, vanilla, dates and cocoa powder in a high-powered blender and start to blend.

2. Drop frozen banana pieces in slowly. Add additional non-dairy milk if needed to reach desired consistency.

Note: Freeze ripe bananas at least 8 hours in advance. Peel bananas and seal in a plastic bag before freezing.

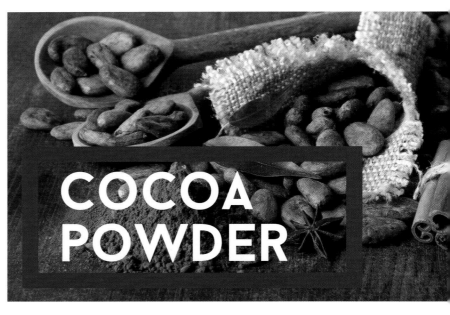

COCOA POWDER

Although many people may use the terms cacao and cocoa interchangeably, they are not the same thing. Both originate from the cacao beans of the Theobroma cacao tree, however cocoa powder is processed at a much higher temperature. To make both powders, cacao beans are fermented, dried and roasted, and then ground to separate and remove the oils. Both cacao and cocoa add a deep and satisfying flavor to dishes on either end of the sweet and savory spectrum – of all the chocolate forms (powder, nibs, butter, liquor), the powder has the highest concentration of unique and healthful phytonutrients known as flavonols.

WHAT MAKES IT SO SPECIAL?

Cocoa is rich in flavonoids and, in particular, flavanols called epicatechin and catechin. These are potent antioxidant and anti-inflammatory agents with a wide range of health benefits. Cocoa supplementation studies in humans suggest that regularly consuming cocoa could lower blood pressure, support healthy arterial function and blood flow, reduce LDL cholesterol and LDL oxidation, and improve insulin sensitivity.[1-4] There is some evidence that cocoa flavanols may also benefit brain function.[5] In general, the highest concentration of beneficial flavanols can be found in darker, less processed chocolate. Look for non-alkalized, pure, unsweetened cocoa powder. Alkalizing (commonly known as "Dutch processing") reduces naturally occurring flavanols, lessening cocoa's potential benefits.

DID YOU KNOW...?

Since cacao powder is produced at a lower temperature, it retains a slightly higher level of heat-sensitive antioxidants. If you're in the market for cocoa powder, stick to plain versions. Cocoa powder "mixes" often contain added sugar or other sweeteners.

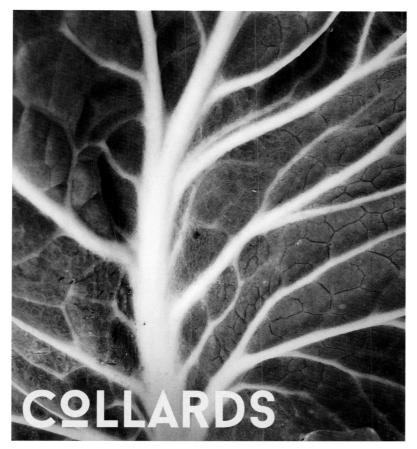

COLLARDS

A popular Southern tradition is eating collard greens and black-eyed peas together on New Year's Day, with the tradition that each food represents a form of wealth, and eating them will bring a prosperous year.

WHAT MAKES THEM SO SPECIAL?

Collards are a dark green leafy cruciferous vegetable that is easy to grow, has a mild taste and is easy to incorporate into your diet in numerous ways. All dark green leafy cruciferous veggies are powerfully cancer protective. Collards provide special nutritional support for three aspects of physiology that are closely connected with cancer development and cancer prevention: the detoxification system, antioxidant defenses, and the balance between pro- and anti-inflammatory substances.[1] Dark cruciferous greens are our real-life "fountain of youth"—they slow aging and protect against all common types of cancer.[2-8]

DID YOU KNOW...?

Collards can be steamed, used in a stir-fry, or eaten raw. They can be used as a healthy wrap, or sliced thin in a salad. A fast four-minute steam makes them soft and pliable enough to use in a multitude of healthful recipes.

CHICKPEA COLLARD WRAPS

SERVES: 3

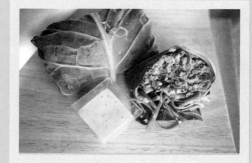

INGREDIENTS

1 can no-salt-added chickpeas, drained
1/2 cup walnuts
1 teaspoon Braggs Liquid Aminos or low-sodium soy sauce
2 teaspoons lemon juice
1 teaspoon Dr. Fuhrman's MatoZest or other no-salt seasoning
6 collard green leaves
1 cup shredded carrots
1 cup shredded red cabbage
1/4 cup chopped red onion
1 avocado, peeled and diced

INSTRUCTIONS

1. In a food processor, pulse the chickpeas, walnuts, Braggs, lemon juice and no-salt seasoning until crumbled and similar in consistency to ground meat.

2. Use a paring knife to shave down the thick stalk of the collard leaves to make them easier to roll.

3. Place an equal amount of the chickpea and walnut mixture on each leaf and top with the carrots, cabbage, onion and avocado. Fold up like a burrito.

If desired, serve with a no-salt, no-oil salad dressing.

CORN

The history of sweet corn, also called maize, began about 9,000 years ago. Scientists have used DNA evidence to trace the timeline of selective breeding – over thousands of years – that turned an almost unrecognizable plant called teosinte (with just a few kernels) first into maize and then into the sweet corn we are familiar with today.

WHAT MAKES IT SO SPECIAL?

Corn is a rich source of ferulic acid, an antioxidant that fights cancer-causing free radicals. In laboratory studies, ferulic acid reduces the growth and proliferation of cancer cells, and also has anti-inflammatory effects when tested on white blood cells.[1] Unlike many other phytochemicals, cooking actually increases the amount of usable ferulic acid in sweet corn – by more than 500 percent. In fact, the total antioxidant activity in corn increases after cooking.[2] In addition, corn is a good source of B vitamins, including thiamin, niacin, folate, and pantothenic acid.

Among grains, corn is especially rich in resistant starch.[3] Resistant starch, similar to fiber, increases satiety but is not digested, and is broken down by beneficial gut bacteria into short-chain fatty acids, such as butyrate, which has beneficial effects on intestinal epithelial cells and may also protect against colon cancer.[4]

Only eat corn that is organically grown or that you grow yourself from organic seed. Eating commercial GMO corn may expose you to harmful chemicals, such as glyphosate and formaldehyde.[5, 6]

DID YOU KNOW...?

The long threads found under the husk are called silks. There is one silk strand on the ear for each kernel of corn. The silk comes first; pollination of each individual silk strand results in the development of the kernel.

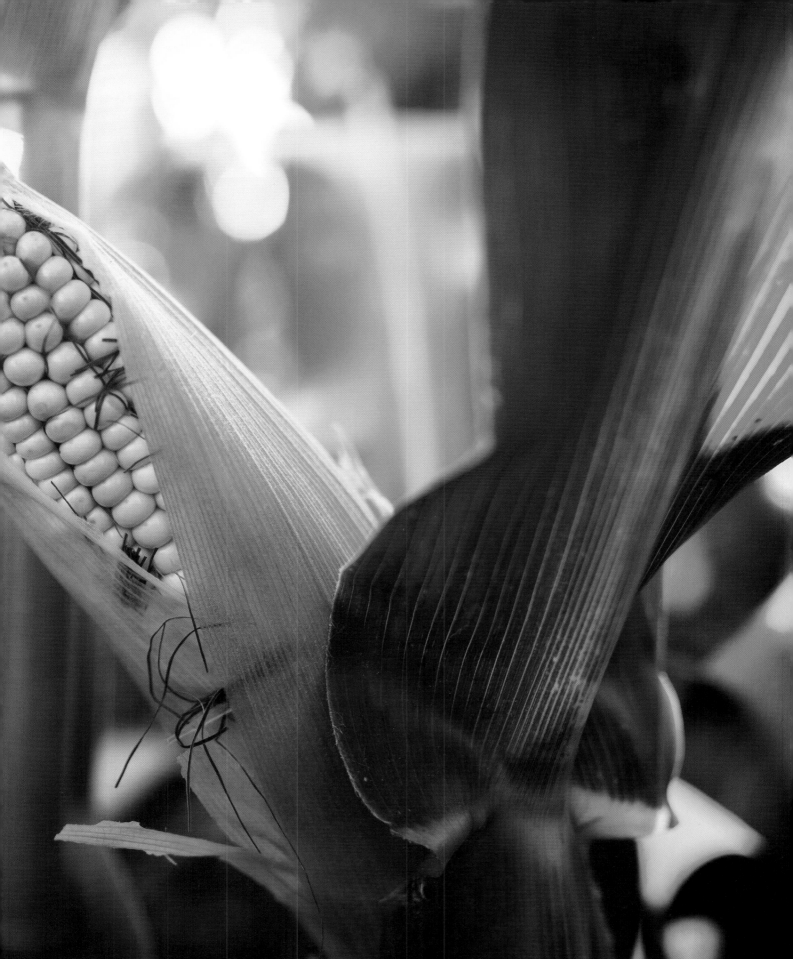

CRANBERRIES

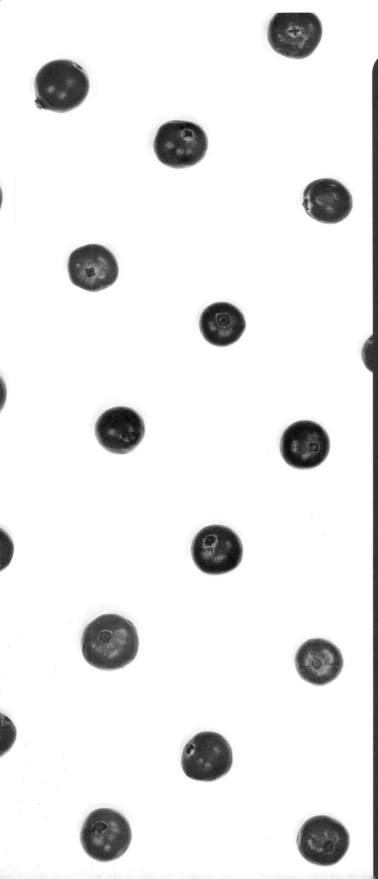

Long before this tart fruit was known as a rich source of vitamin C, fishermen and sailors would take cranberries with them on long journeys, recognizing the berries' value in protecting them from scurvy. Dutch and German settlers first named the fruit "crane berry" because the vines on which they grow resemble the neck, head and bill of a crane.

WHAT MAKES THEM SO SPECIAL?
Enjoying cranberries as part of your diet offers a variety of health benefits, including reduced risk of both cardiovascular disease and cancer. Cranberries are rich in antioxidants called A-type proanthocyanidins, which are not present in most other fruit. A-type proanthocyanidins are known to better prevent the adhesion of bacteria (compared to B-type) and as such, may help in the prevention of tooth decay; they are also thought to provide protection against urinary tract infections.[1,2] Other positive health benefits of eating cranberries include improved insulin sensitivity and vascular function, decreased inflammation and oxidative stress, and improvements in cholesterol levels.[3,4]

It is hard to find dried cranberries that are not heavily sweetened with sugar. Instead, use fresh or frozen and instead of adding sugar, mix and prepare them with other fresh and dried fruits.

DID YOU KNOW...?
Cool trick: Ripe cranberries will actually bounce – try it!

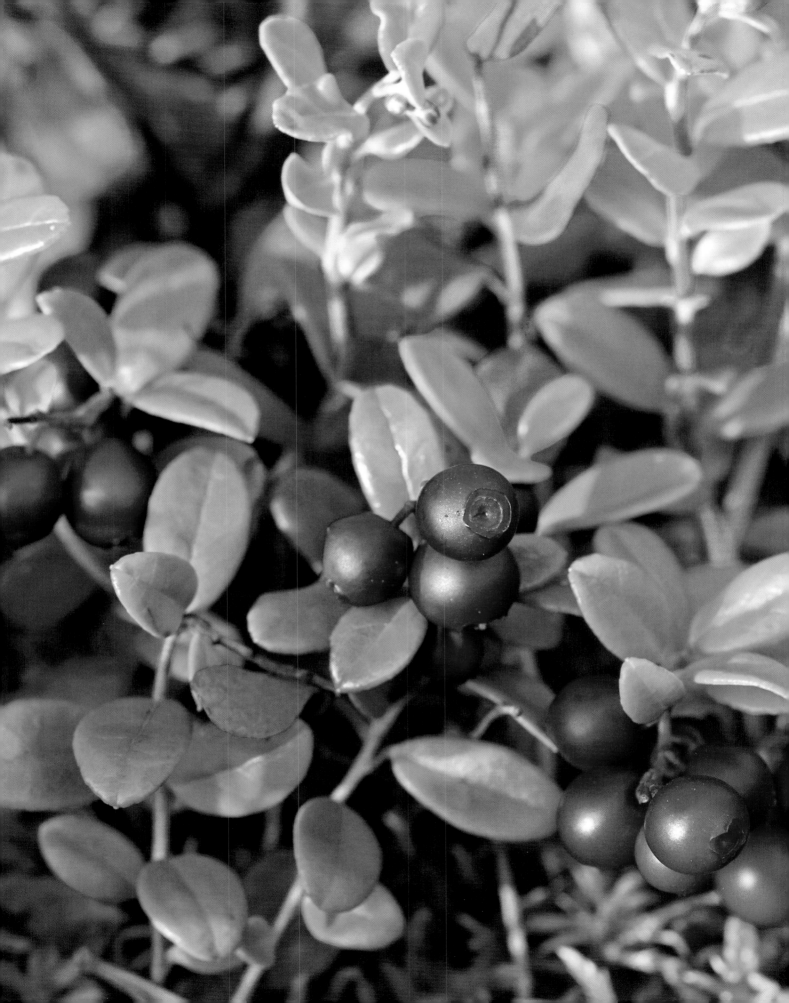

CREAMY CUCUMBER AND ONION SALAD
SERVES: 4

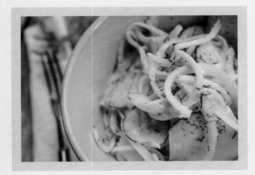

INGREDIENTS
1/2 cup unsweetened soy, hemp or almond milk
1/2 cup raw cashews
1/4 cup white vinegar
1 teaspoon mustard
1 small clove garlic
4 large cucumbers, thinly sliced
1 medium white sweet onion, thinly sliced
1 tablespoon fresh dill or
1 teaspoon dried dill

INSTRUCTIONS
1. Combine non-dairy milk, cashews, vinegar, mustard and garlic in a high-powered blender.

2. Combine cucumbers, onion, and dill and toss with desired amount of dressing.

3. Refridgerate for at least one hour before serving.

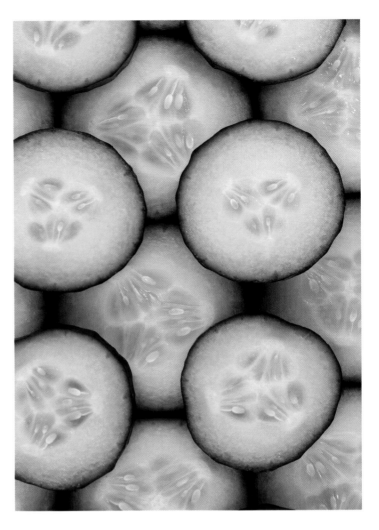

CUCUMBER

The cucumber has the highest water content of any vegetable – over 96 percent, making it a refreshing food to eat on hot summer days. This is probably the origin of the saying, "cool as a cucumber," which usually describes a person who appears calm and collected, despite being in a stressful situation.

WHAT MAKES IT SO SPECIAL?
Cucumbers contain an anti-inflammatory flavonol called fisetin, which has anti-cancer effects in vitro,[1] and may also play a role in brain health. Animal studies suggest that fisetin reduces oxidative stress and inflammation in the brain, leading to protection against age-related cognitive decline and Alzheimer's disease.[2, 3]

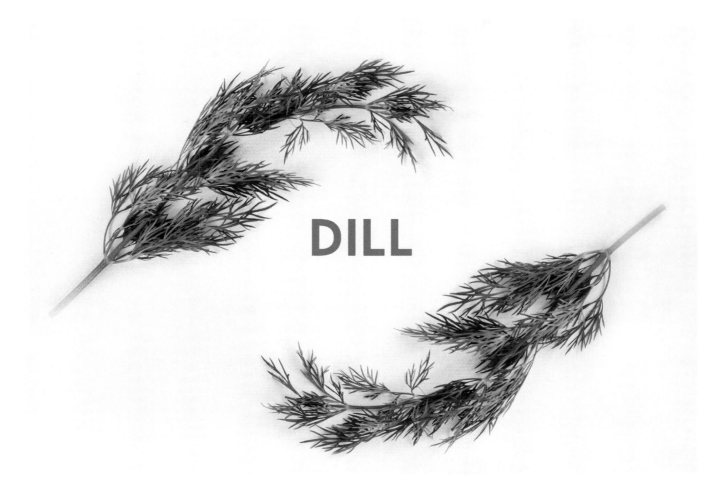

DILL

This age-old herb has been used for its culinary and medicinal properties for at least 5,000 years. Dill is mentioned in medical books from ancient Egypt, where it was used as a medicine, as an aphrodisiac, and as a way to ward off witches.

The dill plant is versatile in that you can use both the leaves and the seeds to provide flavor. "Dill weed" (the term for the plant's leaves) can be used as an herb, while the seeds can be used as a spice. Like many herbs, the seeds and the leaves do have some similarities, but they are not identical. The seeds' flavor is more pungent and some cooks even consider it slightly bitter and reminiscent of camphor; on the other hand, the leaves' flavor is more delicate. Dill seeds also have a characteristic not found in dill weed: their flavor tends to become stronger when heated.

WHAT MAKES IT SO SPECIAL?

Like other deep-green herbs, dill is rich in antioxidants, and fresh herbs have a greater antioxidant activity than dried.[1] Phytochemicals in dill also stimulate the body's natural antioxidant enzymes and detoxification mechanisms.[2] Dill may also reduce the formation of advanced glycation end products (AGEs), harmful substances that contribute to diabetes and its complications.[3] This herb has the ability to impede the growth of microorganisms – one study concluded that dill essential oil could be useful as an eco-friendly antifungal agent.[4]

DID YOU KNOW…?

Try chewing dill seeds – they are thought to help freshen your breath after a meal.

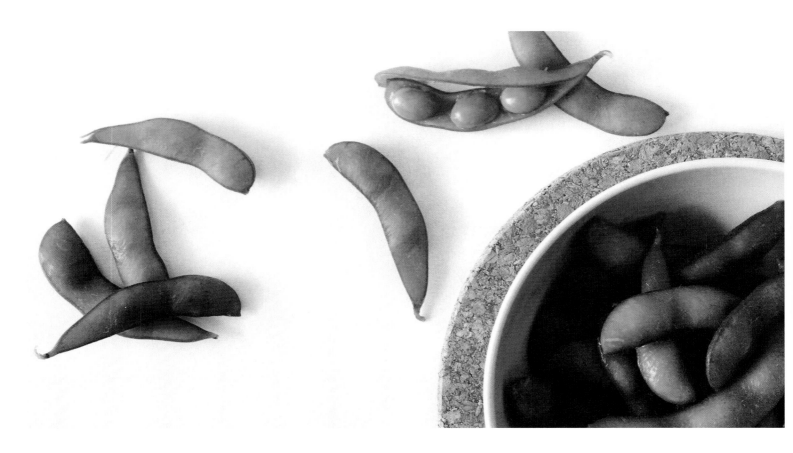

EDAMAME

The word edamame means "beans on a branch" and if you ever saw the plant growing, you'd know it is an accurate description. Native to China, edamame didn't start to catch on in the U.S. until after its health benefits became more widely known. Today, more soybeans are grown in the U.S. than anywhere else in the world.

WHAT MAKES IT SO SPECIAL?

Edamame or boiled soybeans are the healthiest way to eat soy, because it is just the non-processed bean. Eating soy foods has been linked to a decrease in the risk of breast cancer, prostate cancer, lung cancer, colorectal cancer, and cardiovascular disease.[1-6] The health benefits associated with soybeans are thought to be due to plant estrogens called isoflavones. Soy isoflavones have anti-estrogen effects that help to prevent breast cancer but also have a beneficial estrogen-mimicking effect on bone tissue.[1,2,7] Soy isoflavones also have some anti-cancer properties unrelated to estrogen. Edamame is also a good source of calcium, and is high in iron and folate. They are usually purchased frozen and ready to eat, but if cooking them from the raw pods, they should be boiled or steamed for at least 4 minutes or until the color deepens. The pod itself is inedible.

DID YOU KNOW...?

During the Civil War, soybeans were used in place of coffee beans because real coffee was scarce.

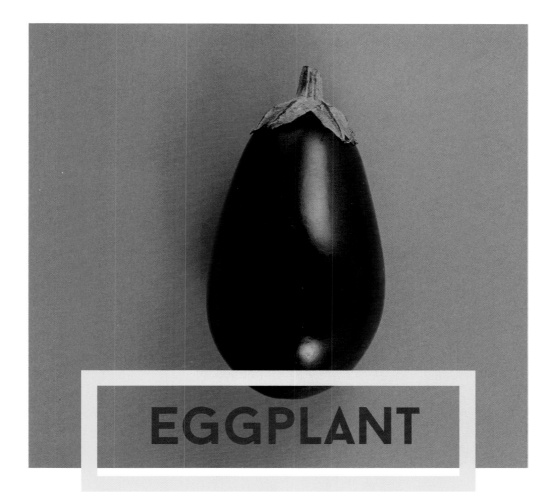

EGGPLANT

The eggplant is a member of the nightshade family, and, like its cousin the tomato, is technically a berry. In the U.K., eggplant is known as aubergine, a word which originates from the ancient language Sanskrit. Eggplant is thought to be native to India, where it is considered to be the King of Vegetables. Eggplant should be cooked, but then can be served in hundreds of delicious ways, both hot or cold. Don't discard the dark nutritious skin of the eggplant. It is great chopped and added to salads and stews.

WHAT MAKES IT SO SPECIAL?

Eggplants are so low in calories, and such a good source of fiber that they are the perfect diet food. The more eggplant you eat, the more weight you lose. However, eggplant is not just a superior "diet" food – it is also associated with a lower risk of cardiovascular disease, diabetes and some cancers. The dark purple skin of eggplants is colored with a flavonoid phytochemical called delphinidin. Studies show nasunin, a derivative of delphinidin also found in eggplant skin, has anti-inflammatory, antioxidant, and anti-angiogenic effects, all of which could contribute to cancer prevention.[1-3]

DID YOU KNOW...?

Eggplant has the highest amount of nicotine of any vegetable, although there is no reason for concern. You would need to eat between 20 to 40 pounds of eggplant to consume the same amount of nicotine that you would get from smoking one cigarette.

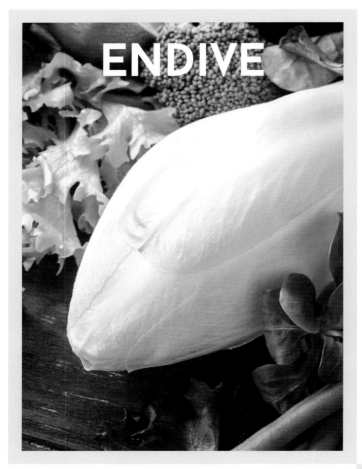

ENDIVE

Escarole is a variety of endive that has been widely cultivated in England since at least the 16th century. It is a member of the leafy chicory family and is very popular in Italian cuisine, especially in the well-known escarole and white bean soup, and as the signature ingredient in "Straciatella," an escarole soup that is commonly made on holidays in Europe.

WHAT MAKES IT SO SPECIAL?

Like other dark leafy greens, escarole is rich in Vitamin K and folate, but more importantly it is a powerhouse of antioxidants and phytochemicals that prolong lifespan and protect against disease. It is an especially good source of multiple carotenoids, including flavonoids, saponins, zeaxanthin and lutein. Escarole has other protective compounds, such as sesquiterpene lactones, and plant sterols, which have anti-inflammatory and anti-tumor effects[1,2]. It is also a great source of minerals like manganese, copper, iron, and potassium.

There are three varieties of endive, a vegetable that is a member of the daisy family. Belgian, the most bitter variety, has small, tightly packed leaves and is grown in complete darkness to prevent it from turning green. Curly is a less bitter variety, and grows in loose, lacey heads. Escarole, the mildest in flavor, has broad, pale green leaves.

WHAT MAKES IT SO SPECIAL?

Endive is a delicious source of folate, vitamin K and the flavonoid kaempferol, which is also found in other leafy greens. Consumption of foods with kaempferol, such as endive, may help to reduce the risk of chronic disease, particularly cancer, by augmenting the body's antioxidant defense against free radicals, which promote cancer's development.[1] Overall, eating foods rich in flavanols such as kaempferol, is associated with reduced risk of ovarian cancer, gastric cancer and breast cancer.[2-4]

DID YOU KNOW...?

It's perfectly fine to pronounce the vegetable's name as "EN-dive," but some purists insist that the Belgian variety is actually "on-DEEV." Hey – you say "po-TAY-to" and I say "po-TAH-to!"

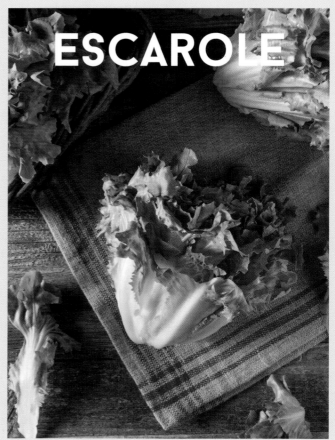

ESCAROLE

FENNEL

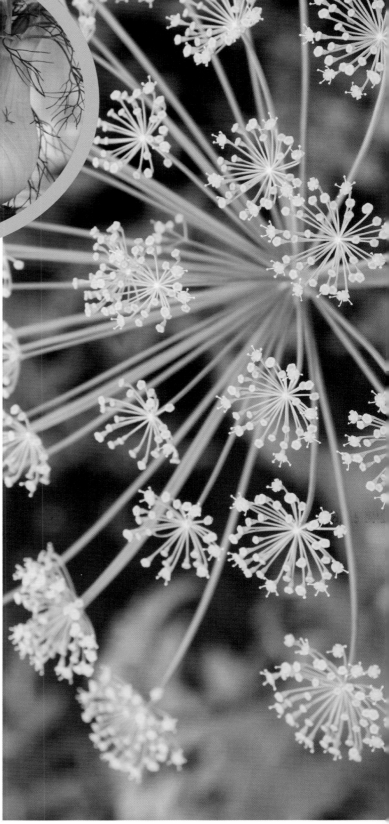

Fennel was revered by the Greeks and the Romans for both its medicinal and culinary properties. English settlers brought the herb with them to the New England colonies, and today it is still found growing on the sites of some of the early settlements. This self-sowing plant grows best during sunny, cool weather.

WHAT MAKES IT SO SPECIAL?

Fennel not only has a delicious licorice flavor, it is also rich in minerals and phytonutrients. The plant and seeds have a reputation as digestive aids,[1] but they also could help to manage symptoms of menopause. Based on new research on a fennel supplement, the plant's phytoestrogens may assist in the management of hot flashes, sleeplessness, vaginal dryness and the anxiety that accompanies menopause.[2] In addition, fennel's major phytochemical, called anethole, has anti-inflammatory and anti-cancer actions.[3, 4]

DID YOU KNOW...?

Fennel can be used both raw and cooked. Every part of fennel is edible, from its feathery fronds to the white bulb. Use the bulb at the bottom of the plant by removing the stalks and slicing the bulb in half, lengthwise. The bulb can be eaten raw and used in salads; the fronds can be used as an herb, and the tough stalks can be added to a vegetable stock or soup.

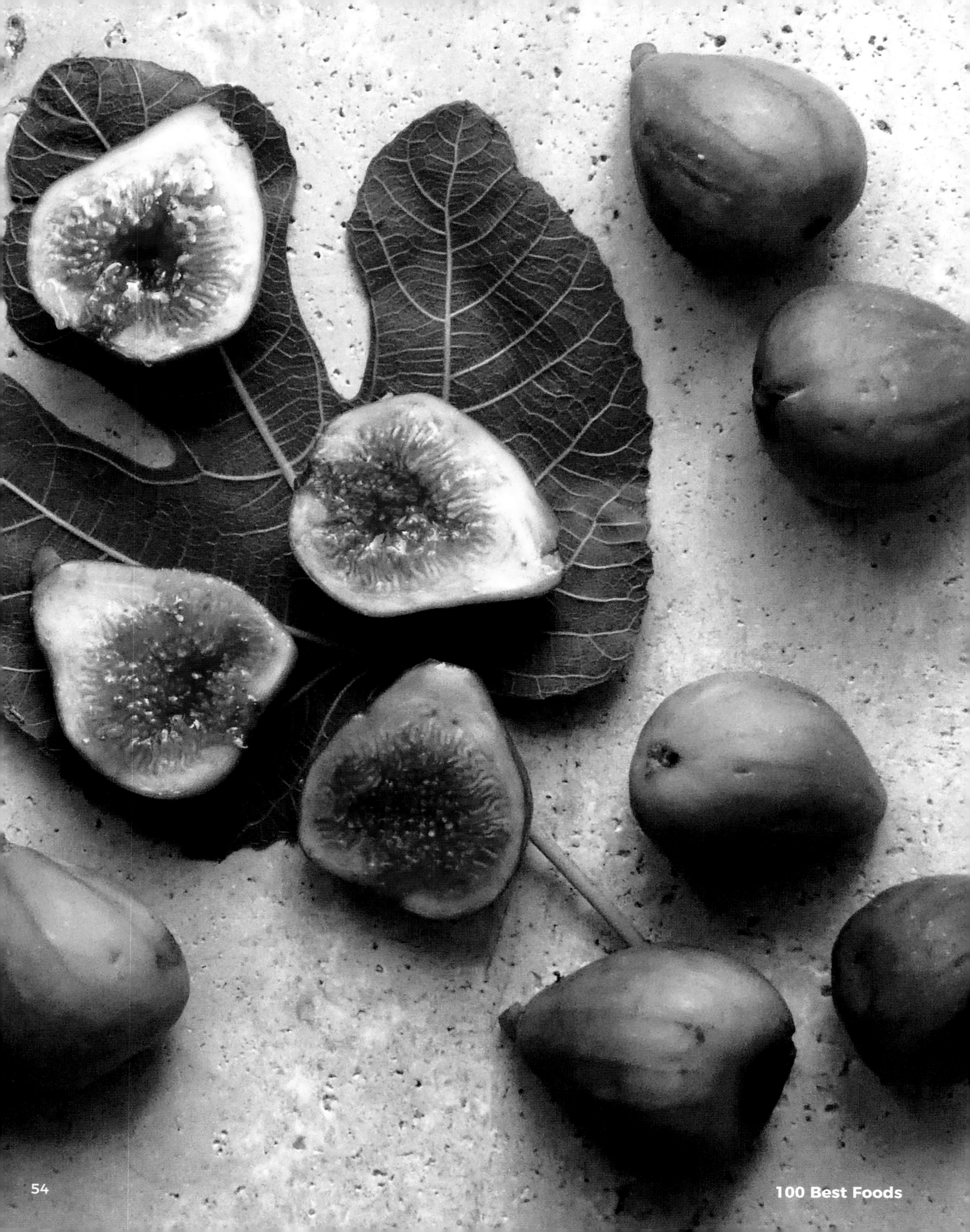

FIGS

Figs were one of the first edible plants cultivated by humans, predating the domestication of wheat and rye by about 1,000 years. Figs were so important to ancient Greeks that they made a law against exporting the trees.

Figs differ dramatically in color and subtly in texture depending upon the variety, of which there are more than one hundred and fifty. Some of the most popular varieties are:

Black Mission: blackish-purple skin and pink flesh

Kadota: green skin and purplish flesh

Calimyrna: greenish-yellow skin and amber flesh

Brown Turkey: purple skin and red flesh

Adriatic: the variety most often used to make fig bars, which has a light green skin and pink-red flesh

WHAT MAKES THEM SO SPECIAL?

The fig is regarded as a superfruit because of its high levels of antioxidants and phytochemicals, total and soluble fiber, magnesium, calcium, and potassium.[1] The fiber and concentrated micronutrients can help lower blood pressure, lower cholesterol levels, slow the absorption of calories and provide a feeling of satiety.[2-4]

Figs are rich in polyphenols which help combat oxidative stress.[1, 5, 6] Even the leaves of the fig tree are edible, and fig leaves may help reduce glucose for people with diabetes.[7]

Figs are fragile, so many delicious species are not sold commercially. They are simple to grow in the southern states, but also can be easily grown in northern regions when planted in large pots that can be moved indoors, or placed in a shed or in the garage for the coldest winter months.

Small trees can produce lots of fruit when still just a few feet tall, so they are fun trees to cultivate – you don't have to wait five years or more to get delicious fruit.

FUDGY FIG BITES
SERVES: 10

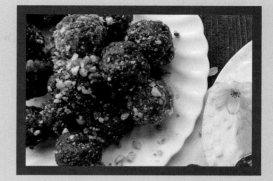

INGREDIENTS
2 cups unsulfured dried figs, stems removed
1/2 cup chopped walnuts
1/2 cup chopped raw cashews or almonds
1 teaspoon vanilla bean powder
1/4 cup natural cocoa powder

INSTRUCTIONS
1. Chop figs into small pieces. and place in a food processor

2. Add remaining ingredients and continue to process until the mixture forms a paste and begins to adhere together.

3. Form into small balls.

If desired, roll in additional cocoa powder or chopped nuts. Makes approximately 30 pieces.

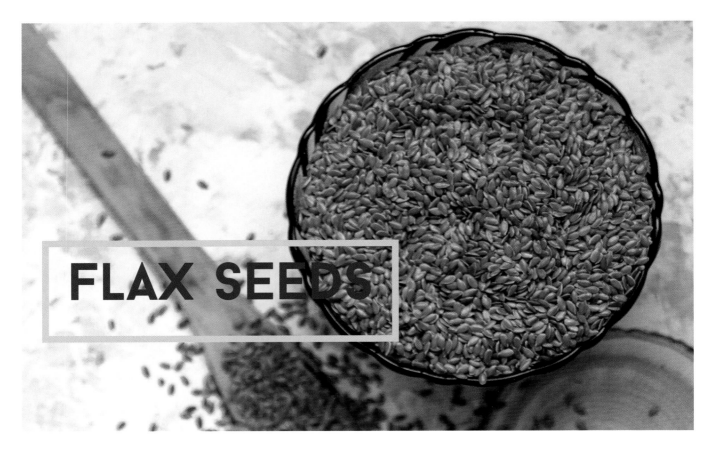

FLAX SEEDS

Flax seeds were cultivated in Babylon as early as 3000 B.C. By the 8th century, King Charlemagne believed so strongly in the health benefits of flax seed that he passed laws requiring his subjects to consume it.

WHAT MAKES THEM SO SPECIAL?

Supplementing the diet with flax seeds has been shown to lower systolic and diastolic blood pressure in many human studies. [1] A unique feature of flax seeds is a group of nutrients called lignans, which have powerful antioxidant and anti-estrogenic properties and help in preventing breast and prostate cancer, as well as other types of cancer. [2-4] In one interesting study, women who were diagnosed with breast cancer were placed into a flax group or a control group for about one month, until surgery. Tumor tissue compared between diagnosis and surgery revealed significant apoptosis (cell death) and reduced proliferation of cancer cells in the flax group in that short time.[5] Scientists have also discovered that flax seeds may protect healthy tissues and organs from the harmful effects of radiation. Dietary flax seed given to mice protected lung tissues before exposure to radiation, and also significantly reduced damage after exposure. When incorporating flax seeds into your diet, remember to always eat them ground. According to the Flax Council of Canada, ground flax seeds provide more nutritional benefits than whole flax seeds. They have a very tough outer shell that may not be broken down when you chew. Your stomach acid is also unable to break through the shell and whole flax seeds may pass through your gut completely intact. Grinding flax seeds opens them up and makes them easier for your body to digest, so you can benefit from all of the essential nutrients.

DID YOU KNOW...?

The fibers in the stem of the flax plant are used to make linen – a thread that is stronger than cotton.

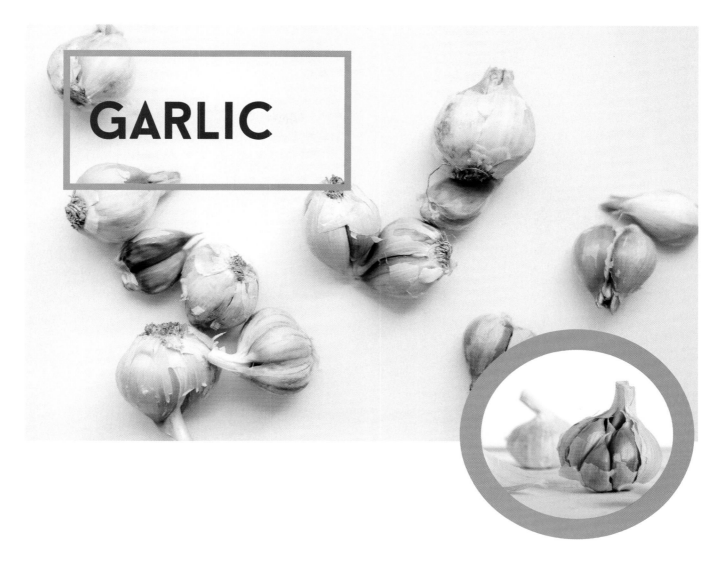

GARLIC

Ancient Egyptians worshiped it, and placed clay models of garlic bulbs in the tomb of Tutankhamen. Hippocrates (460 B.C. to 370 B.C.) was said to have used garlic to treat cancerous tumors.

WHAT MAKES IT SO SPECIAL

Garlic's health benefits affect our cardiovascular system, immune system, inflammatory response and detoxification processes.[1, 2] Garlic aids cardiovascular health by slowing the production of cholesterol, and reducing oxidation of LDL cholesterol and platelet aggregation.[3, 4] Garlic's signature organosulfur compounds have cancer-fighting effects, and greater intake of garlic is linked to a reduced risk of several different cancers, including esophageal, colorectal, breast, and prostate cancers.[2, 5]

Do not store garlic in the refrigerator as this encourages sprouting. Do not freeze; it will change the flavor and consistency of the garlic.

PREPARATION

The most nutritious way to cook garlic is to chop, slice, mince or crush it raw, and then add the crushed garlic to your wok, soup or stew.

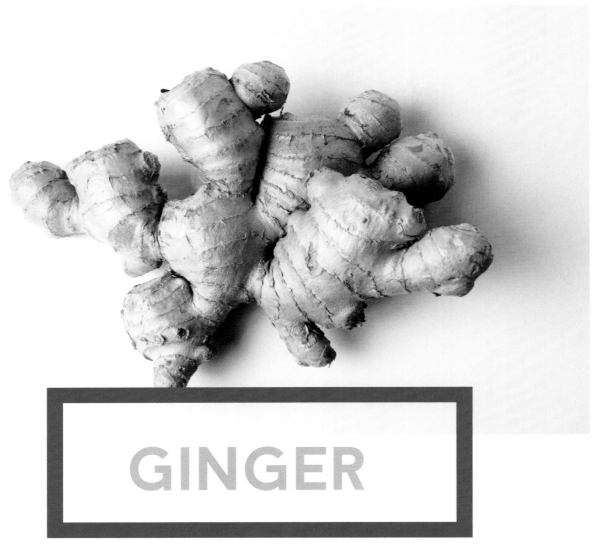

GINGER

Throughout history, ginger has been prized as a digestive aid. Confucius wrote in circa 500 B.C. of never being without ginger when he ate; during the Revolutionary War, ginger's stomach-soothing properties made it an important part of the American soldiers' diet.

WHAT MAKES IT SO SPECIAL?

Ginger contains a number of unique and powerful anti-inflammatory compounds called gingerols, which have been shown in mice to prevent carcinogenic activity in the colon that can lead to colorectal cancer. Many in vitro studies show anti-cancer effects of gingerols.[1-3] Several studies suggest ginger is an effective treatment for nausea, because of its effect on the gastrointestinal system and nervous system. These studies have been done on pregnant women and people with motion sickness.[4] There are also interesting studies on ginger as a treatment for pain. In patients with osteoarthritis, menstrual pain, and migraines, studies show that supplemental ginger successfully reduces pain.[5-8] When purchasing ginger, look for rhizomes (ginger roots) that are heavy for their size, with firm skin and a spicy fragrance. Slice ginger perpendicular to its fibers to eliminate any stringiness.

DID YOU KNOW...?

Gingerbread "people" cookies have their roots in international relations. In the 16th century, England's Queen Elizabeth I liked to present her important visitors with gingerbread men decorated to look like themselves.

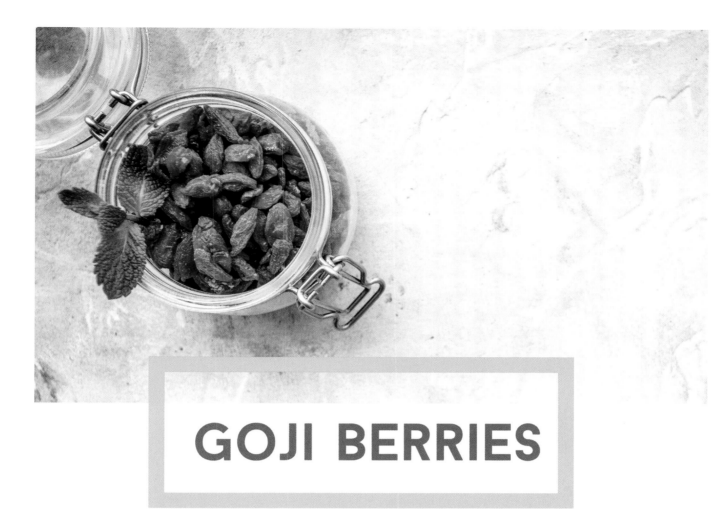

GOJI BERRIES

Goji berries have been used for thousands of years in China and in other Asian countries as both a food and as a medicinal herb to treat diabetes and improve eyesight. Legend has it that goji berries, or wolfberries as they are also known, provide a pathway to the Fountain of Youth. Lately, this brightly-colored berry has been touted as a superfood.

WHAT MAKES THEM SO SPECIAL?

Small but mighty, goji berries are packed with vitamin C, are rich in carotenoid and flavonoid antioxidants, and are high in fiber. Their major carotenoid, zeaxanthin, is one of the two carotenoids known to protect the retina against light damage.[1] In vitro and animal studies suggest goji berry phytochemicals activate the body's natural antioxidant system and detoxification enzymes, and help keep the immune system working properly.[2] Plus, several studies in humans have shown that consumption of goji berry juice or goji berry extract improves immune function and markers of antioxidant capacity.[3]

DID YOU KNOW...?

Sun-dried Goji berries are much more popular than fresh Goji berries (which are available in specialty stores) because they retain the same nutrients, but have a more concentrated flavor.

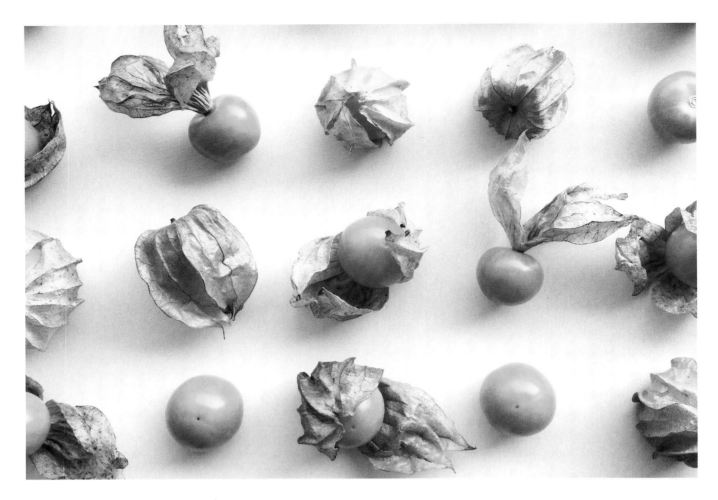

GOOSEBERRIES

Though the origin of the name "gooseberry" is unclear, it has been a popular fruit in Europe, Asia and Northern Africa since at least the 16th century. The fruit grows on low, thorny bushes that can yield both tart and sweet berries. The Indian gooseberry (known as amla) which is light green and very sour, has traditionally been used in Ayurvedic medicine.

WHAT MAKES THEM SO SPECIAL?

Gooseberries come in a wide range of flavors, colors and shapes. The American and European varieties can be yellow, green, red and black; oval, round, or elongated; and sweet or tart. The fruit contains antioxidant flavones, polyphenolics and anthocyanins, which offer protection against cancer and inflammation. One cup of gooseberries provides 26 percent of your daily fiber requirement, and 69 percent of your required vitamin C. The berries also provide lots of carotenoids, B vitamins, and minerals. In vitro studies on Indian gooseberries have indicated that extracts of the berry block proliferation and promote cell death in breast, ovarian, cervical, and other types of cancer cells.[1] These berries contain a number of phytochemicals known to have antioxidant and anti-inflammatory effects, such as ellagic acid and quercetin.[1] Study participants who supplemented with gooseberry powder daily reduced fasting blood glucose, triglycerides, and LDL cholesterol.[2, 3]

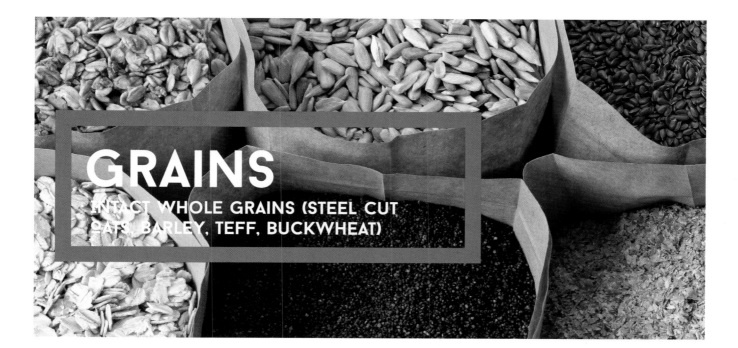

GRAINS
INTACT WHOLE GRAINS (STEEL CUT OATS, BARLEY, TEFF, BUCKWHEAT)

Delicious and chewy, intact whole grains have many nutritional advantages over refined grains or even whole grain flour products. Unrefined whole grains have not had their natural bran and germ removed, so they retain more beneficial fiber and resistant starch than more processed grains. Eating these grains whole (and cooked in water) limits their glycemic effects. Get in touch with the Old World by substituting nutritious, ancient grains for white rice, white potatoes and white pasta.

WHAT MAKES THEM SO SPECIAL?

Intact whole grains are slowly absorbed and gradually metabolized, while grains that are refined (like white rice) or processed into flour are quickly absorbed, leading to spikes in blood sugar and insulin. Even whole grain flours, typically baked into bread, are not as healthful as intact whole grains cooked in water. Collectively, research has shown that those who include fiber-rich foods like whole grains in their diet are less likely to develop diabetes, colon cancer, and heart disease.[1, 2] The viscous fiber in **oats** is especially helpful for keeping cholesterol down.[3] **Steel cut oats** (sometimes called Irish or Scottish oats) are the minimally processed version and best choice of oatmeal: thick pieces of chopped oats are digested more slowly and have a smaller effect on blood sugar than old-fashioned rolled oats and more highly processed instant oatmeal. **Barley** comes in different types, which are not interchangeable: Pearled barley is the most common kind, but it's the "white rice" of barley – it's not a whole grain. There are two types of whole grain barley: hulled barley, in which the outer hull has been removed but the grain itself and its bran layer remains intact; and hulless barley, a variety which never forms a hull. Either may also be called barley groats. **Buckwheat**, although technically not a grain but a pseudocereal, is a nutritional powerhouse, containing high levels of phytonutrients, particularly the flavonoid rutin, which has anti-inflammatory and glucose-lowering effects.[4, 5] If the buckwheat has been roasted (kasha) it is good to go, otherwise you can lightly toast the raw buckwheat in a shallow saucepan to firm its texture and enhance its flavor. After toasting, boil the buckwheat using a ratio of 1 cup buckwheat to 1.5 cups water. **Teff** is a cereal grass that is a staple food in its native Ethiopia, a country that grows 90 percent of the world's supply. The small seeds of this gluten-free grain have a nutty flavor and are rich in nutrients – one cup of cooked teff contains 7.1 grams of fiber, 9.8 grams of protein and 29 percent of the daily requirement of iron.

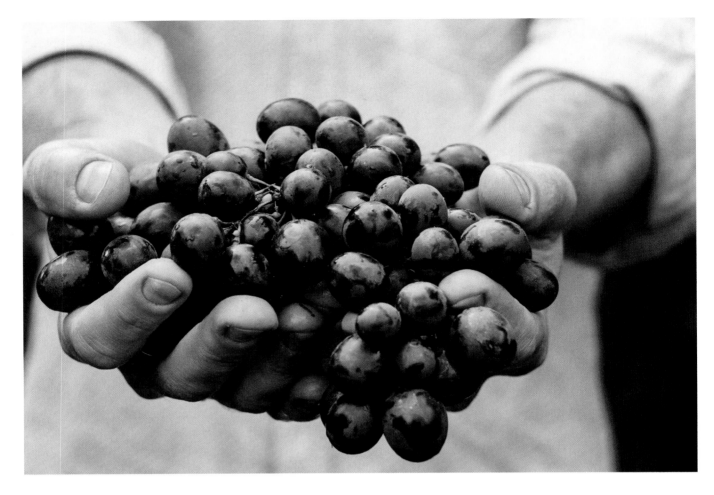

GRAPES

Grapes were first introduced to America by Spanish explorers approximately 300 years ago, although the cultivation of grapes started over 8,000 years ago. Eating grapes rather than drinking them was not recorded in history until the early 16th century, when King Francois I of France regularly ate grapes for dessert. There are over 8,000 grape varieties from about 60 different species. Raisins are dried sweet grapes, dried naturally by being left out in the sun.

WHAT MAKES THEM SO SPECIAL?

Red grape skins are known for their resveratrol content. Resveratrol is a polyphenol that generated research interest for its ability to mimic the longevity-promoting effects of calorie restriction in animal studies. Clinical trials often use high doses of supplemental resveratrol which would be unreasonable to get in one's diet, but some have used whole grapes in more usual amounts, with positive results. One clinical trial found participants who ate whole red grapes daily for eight weeks increased their blood antioxidant capacity and reduced total and LDL cholesterol levels. Another trial found that grape powder increased anti-inflammatory markers.[1,2] In patients with colon cancer, grape powder showed cancer-preventive effects in their healthy colon cells.[3]

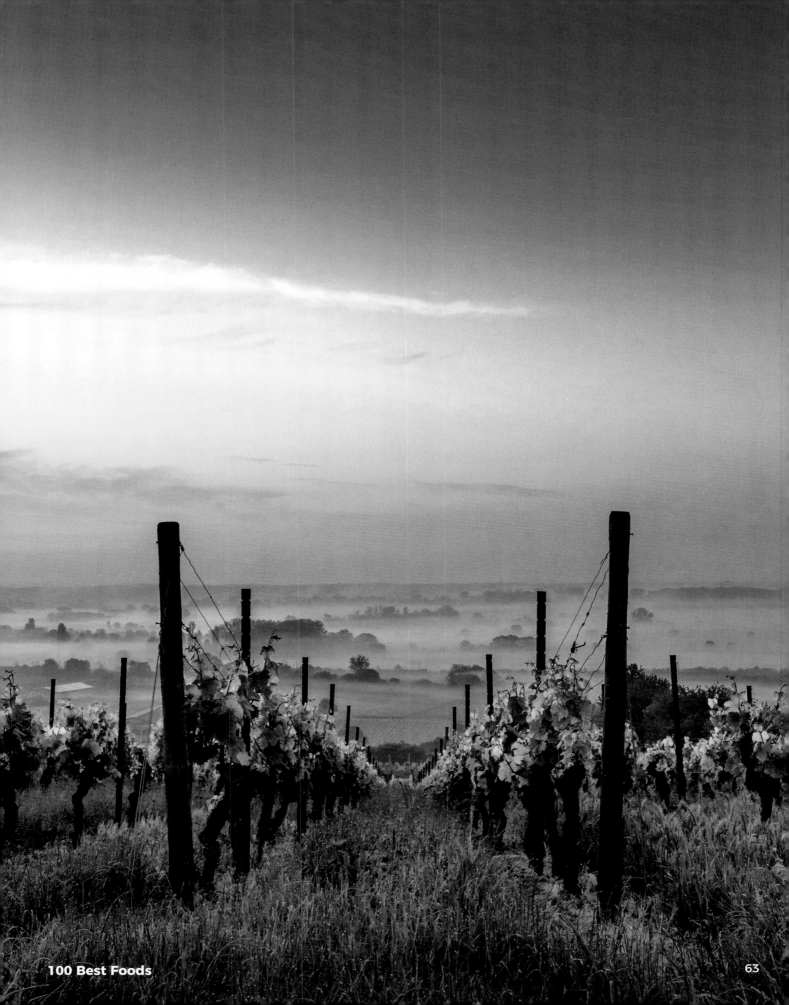

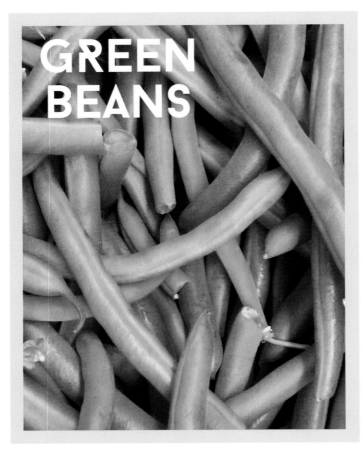

GREEN BEANS

Green tea originated in China, where it was used for medicinal purposes before becoming a popular daily drink. Enjoy it plain, since there is evidence that adding milk (dairy or not) to green tea may blunt some of its benefit.[1,2]

WHAT MAKES IT SO SPECIAL?
Drinking green tea regularly has been linked to reduced risk of heart disease, stroke, lung cancer, breast cancer, prostate cancer, diabetes and all-cause mortality.[3-11] It is also thought to help prevent or slow brain aging.[12,13] Green tea is especially rich in the antioxidant polyphenol epigallocatechin-3-gallate (EGCG). Increasing evidence has suggested that EGCG exhibits anti-inflammatory and antioxidant effects. Although EGCG is present to some degree in all teas, it is found in almost no other foods.[14]

DID YOU KNOW...?
Green tea's beneficial antioxidant EGCG is released slowly, so a longer steep time is better.[15] If you prefer iced tea, be aware that antioxidant activity was found to be similar in green teas steeped in hot water for seven minutes, compared to those steeped in cold water for two hours.[16]

Green beans are called by many different names: French beans, fine beans, string beans, or even squeaky beans. There are approximately 150 varieties of green beans throughout the world, and they come in all shapes and colors – even purple. Green beans are like a cross between a green vegetable and a bean, making them unique in the plant kingdom.

WHAT MAKES THEM SO SPECIAL?
Green beans are low in calories and rich in nutrients, at only 45 calories a cup. Two cups supply 5 grams of protein, as well as omega-3 fatty acids (ALA). They contain a full spectrum of carotenoids, including the unusual and valuable violaxanthin and neoxanthin. They are also rich in silicon and vitamin K, which are nutrients that support bone health.[1,2] Steam green beans for only 5 to 8 minutes to best retain their nutrients.

DID YOU KNOW...?
Every year, on the last Saturday in July, the city of Blairsville, Georgia holds its Green Bean Festival. The celebration includes cooking contests, canning plant tours, beauty pageants and other activities that showcase the vegetable.

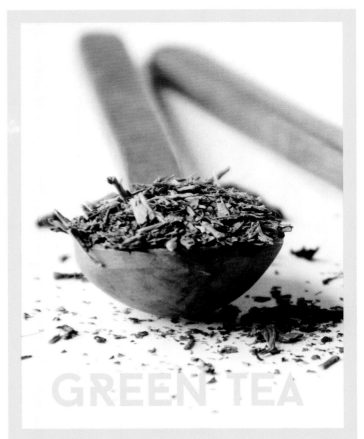

GREEN TEA

HAZELNUTS

Whether you call them filberts, cobnuts or hazels, the hazelnut is popular throughout the world, and has been a source of food for thousands of years. Traditionally, the tree was a symbol of marriage, abundance, wealth, and family happiness.

WHAT MAKES THEM SO SPECIAL?

These rustic brown nuts are a good source of fiber and also contain phytosterols which have multiple health effects, including reducing LDL cholesterol. Indeed, multiple clinical trials adding hazelnuts to the diet have reported reductions in LDL cholesterol.[1, 2] Hazelnuts also provide antioxidant phytochemicals, such as various vitamin E fragments, proanthocyanidins and flavonoids, and there is evidence from human studies that hazelnuts help prevent the oxidation of LDL cholesterol.[2-4]

DID YOU KNOW...?

In ancient Rome, hazel branches were used as torches during the wedding night, as they were thought to ensure fertility and a happy marriage.

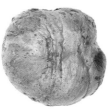

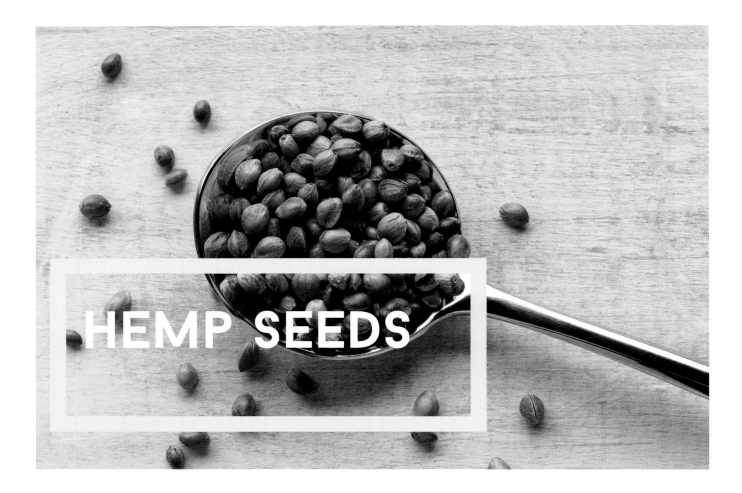

HEMP SEEDS

These tiny members of the cannabis plant have wide-ranging health benefits. Although hemp and marijuana are both members of the same plant species, hemp seeds won't make you high, because hemp naturally has almost no THC (Tetrahydrocannabinol), the active ingredient in marijuana. Hemp flowers contain just 0.3 percent THC, which is about 30 times less than the least-potent marijuana. This means that it's impossible to get high from hemp, although many people have tried!

WHAT MAKES THEM SO SPECIAL?

Hemp seeds, along with chia seeds, flax seeds and walnuts, are the richest whole food sources of the omega-3 fatty acid, alpha-linolenic acid (ALA). ALA is converted to DHA and EPA, the omega-3s that are crucial for brain health.[1] Hemp seeds also provide plant sterols, iron, and vitamin E.[2] The seeds are composed of about 30 percent fat and 25 percent protein,[3] and can provide a whole food, nutrient-rich boost of protein for athletes who may need extra. Hemp seeds are also rich in arginine, an amino acid that helps to keep blood pressure down.[3]

DID YOU KNOW...?

The hemp plant successfully competes with weeds, and problems with pests are mostly insignificant – this means that pesticides and herbicides are largely unnecessary for growing hemp seeds.[4]

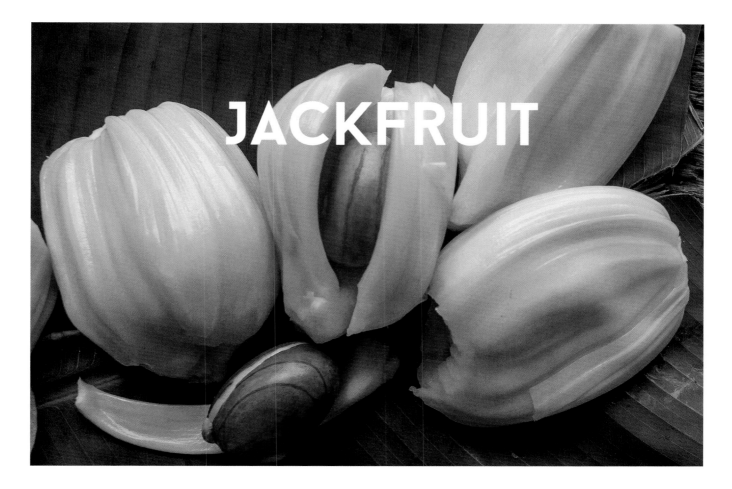

JACKFRUIT

Jackfruit is the largest tree fruit in the world. The fruit grows on both the branches and the tree's trunk. At maturity the fruits fall to the ground, but you better not be under the tree when that happens, because mature jackfruit can weigh anywhere from 10 to 50 pounds. Growers often harvest it early to avoid having the large fruits fall on top of anyone. The edible parts of the fruit are the bright yellow "bulbs" just beneath the rind. Its seeds can also be dried and eaten. Packaged, unripe jackfruit has become a popular and healthful alternative to pork in tacos, wraps, and sandwiches. Ripe jackfruit can be found in Asian markets and in some grocery stores, and it is also available frozen and dried.

WHAT MAKES IT SO SPECIAL?

This almost prehistoric-looking fruit is nutrient-dense, and contains a special protein called jacalin, a plant lectin. Plant lectins recognize certain carbohydrates, and some lectins recognize a carbohydrate found on the surface of cancerous cells, and may help prevent cancer development by blocking the proliferation of those cells.[1,2] Dietary jacalin in particular has been shown to inhibit the development of colon cancer in mice.[3] In addition to jacalin, Jackfruit also provides lots of beta-carotene, potassium, magnesium, riboflavin, vitamin B6, and vitamin C.

DID YOU KNOW...?

Jackfruit has a distinctive sweet smell, and the riper it gets, the stronger its smell. When purchasing it fresh, let the skin get brown and give in to pressure, until it almost smells rotten. That increases the flavor and sweetness of the bulbs inside. The fruits are so big, that you may have to freeze some of the fruit if you don't have a big enough family to eat all the freshly harvested bulbs within a week.

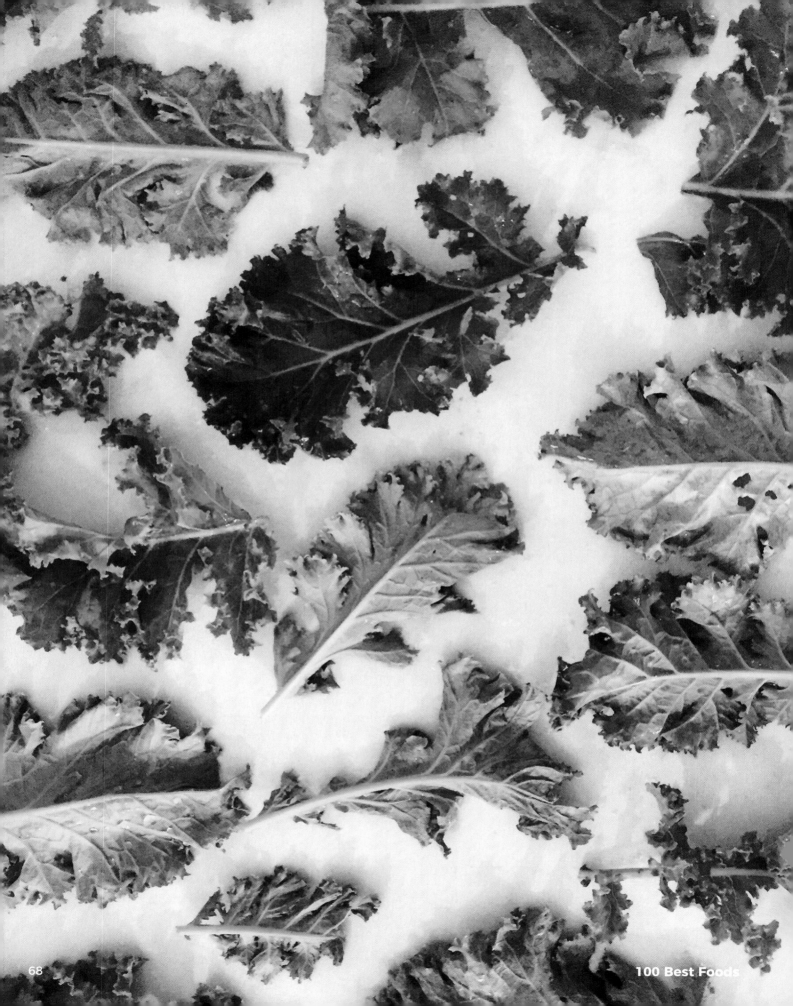

KALE

With antioxidant carotenoids and flavonoids, plus ample amounts of vitamin C, folate, calcium and iron, kale is king of the nutritional kingdom. While most of us are familiar with the curly or flat green varieties, kale can range in color from blue-green to red or purple. Though known primarily as a cool weather crop, frost actually makes kale sweeter.

WHAT MAKES IT SO SPECIAL?

Kale contains substances that protect against inflammation, reduce oxidation, and prevent damage to DNA – properties that protect against cardiovascular disease and cancer.[1, 2] When cruciferous greens are chewed (or crushed before being consumed), isothiocyanates (ITCs) are formed. These ITCs are a significant factor in the reduced risk of cancer, cardiovascular disease, as well as death from all causes observed with greater comsuption of cruciferous vegetables.[3] A one cup serving of cooked kale supplies 94 mg of calcium (of which 50 percent is absorbable). This is a high fractional absorption for calcium; by comparison, that figure is only 30 percent for cow's milk.[4] Kale can be eaten raw in salads (remove the tough middle stems), or cooked.

DID YOU KNOW...?

Kale and other plants in the Brassica family produce flowers that are in the shape of a cross. For that reason, these plants are referred to as 'crucifers' or more commonly, cruciferous.

CALIFORNIA CREAMED KALE
SERVES: 4

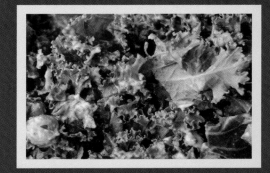

INGREDIENTS
2 bunches kale, leaves removed from tough stems
1 cup raw cashews (or 1/2 cup raw cashews and 1/2 cup hemp seeds)
3/4 cup unsweetened soy, hemp or almond milk
1/4 cup dehydrated onion flakes
1 tablespoon Dr. Fuhrman's VegiZest or nutritional yeast (or other no-salt seasoning blend, adjusted to taste)

INSTRUCTIONS
1. Place kale in a large steamer pot. Steam 6-8 minutes or until soft.

2. Meanwhile, place remaining ingredients in a high-powered blender and blend until smooth.

3. Place kale in colander and press to remove the excess water. In a bowl, coarsely chop and mix kale with the cream sauce.

Note: Sauce may be used with broccoli, spinach, or other steamed vegetables.

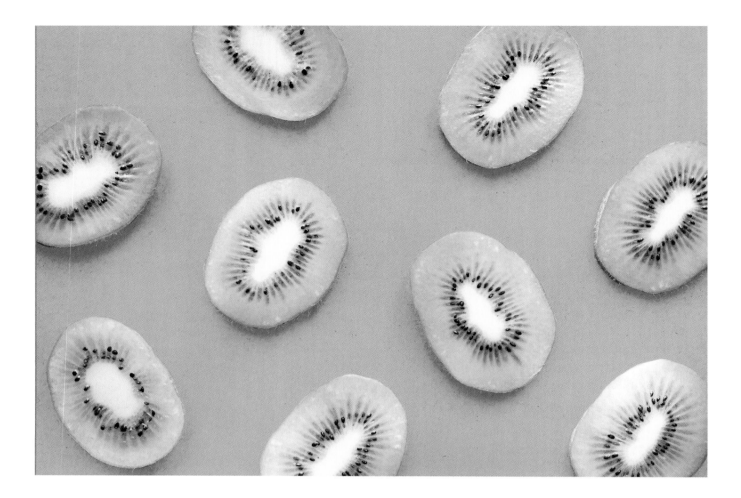

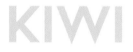

KIWI

Originally known as a Chinese Gooseberry, this fruit grows on long vines – up to 33 feet! It was renamed kiwifruit by New Zealanders for its resemblance to the rounded body and fuzzy brown plumage of their native (flightless) kiwi bird.

WHAT MAKES IT SO SPECIAL?

By weight, a kiwi contains two times more vitamin C than oranges. Kiwis also contain phytochemicals with strong antioxidant potential and are a rich source of vitamin K, vitamin E and folate. Preliminary research in humans suggests eating kiwis may benefit immune function, sleep quality, antioxidant defenses, and digestive health.[1-4] Kiwi is a smart fruit choice for those with diabetes, as its high amount of soluble and insoluble fiber contributes to its low- to moderate-glycemic load rating, meaning that it does not rapidly raise blood glucose levels.

DID YOU KNOW...?

Kiwifruits should be eaten soon after cutting, since they contain enzymes that act as a food tenderizer, with the ability to further tenderize the kiwifruit itself and make it overly soft. Consequently, if you are adding kiwifruit to fruit salad, you should do so at the last minute to prevent the other fruits from becoming too soggy.

KOHLRABI

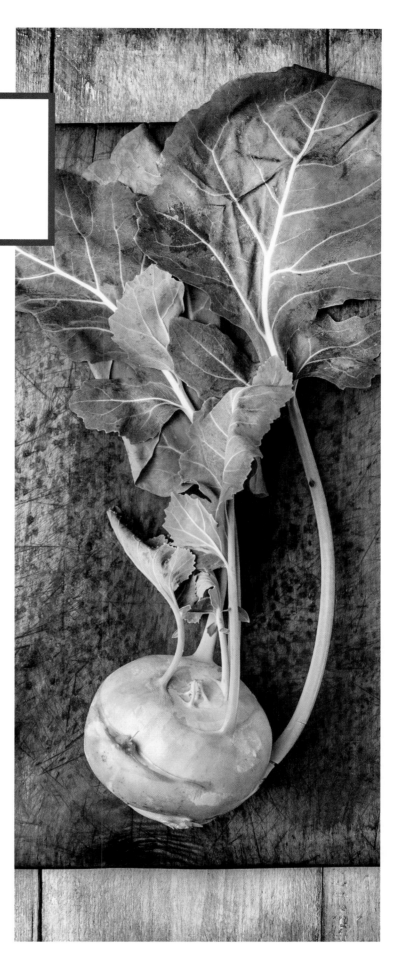

Although not widely known in the U.S., kohlrabi is grown here. Kohlrabi comes in light green (sometimes called white) and purple (called red) colors. It is cruciferous, a relative of cabbage, and has been gaining more and more recognition.

WHAT MAKES IT SO SPECIAL?

Kohlrabi is a good source of fiber and micronutrients such as vitamin B6 and potassium. One cup of kohlrabi contains more than a day's worth of vitamin C.[1]

As a cruciferous vegetable, Kohlrabi produces cancer-fighting isothiocyanates (ITCs) when they are chopped (which is best done before heating) or chewed (when eaten raw). Extracts of red and green kohlrabi have been shown to reduce the production of inflammatory compounds in white blood cells, and to produce beneficial effects on insulin signaling that may help to protect against type 2 diabetes.[2]

DID YOU KNOW...?

You can eat the leaves of the plant and the bulb either raw in salads or, if desired, cooked, to soften more.

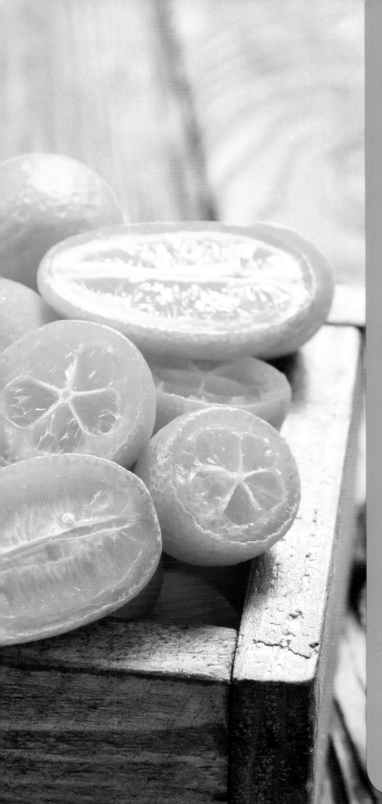

KUMQUATS

The word "kumquat" means "golden orange" in Mandarin. The fruits are native to China, where they are considered a symbol of prosperity. Nagami kumquats, the type we mostly see in the U.S., look like tiny, oval-shaped oranges and are tart. Meiwa kumquats are rounder and sweeter. Mandarinquats, a cross between a mandarin orange and a kumquat, are larger, teardrop-shaped and sweeter than the more common Nagami kumquats. The Meiwa tree stays small and can grow nicely in a pot in your living room, or it can be kept outside and easily moved indoors or in the garage in colder weather. I recommend having at least one Meiwa kumquat plant in the house.

WHAT MAKES THEM SO SPECIAL?

Small in size, but big in health benefits, the flesh of kumquats is rich in vitamin C, while the edible skin contains a number of flavonoids and phenolic acids.[1] Kumquat extract has been shown to inhibit proliferation and promote cell death in prostate cancer cells.[2] There is also some evidence that kumquat extract has blood glucose-lowering activity.[3]

Although they look like tiny oranges, kumquats are classified in a separate genus from citrus fruits like lemons, limes, and grapefruits.[3] What makes them unique is the favorable dose of limonene, in the skin of the fruit, that protects our skin from aging, wrinkling and from skin cancer.

LENTILS

Shaped like a lens, thus the name, lentils have been a source of sustenance for our ancestors since prehistoric times. They are frequently mentioned in the Bible, most notably in the Genesis story of Esau and Jacob. The firstborn, Esau, sold his birthright to his twin brother Jacob in exchange for lentil stew.

WHAT MAKES THEM SO SPECIAL?

Small in size, lentils are big in protecting your health owing, in part, to their high micronutrient and high fiber content. Eating legumes (such as lentils and beans) regularly may lower the risk of heart disease, as these fiber-rich foods are known to reduce cholesterol levels.[1] Adding lentils to the diet has been found to reduce blood pressure and measures of insulin resistance.[2] The high-fiber content of lentils also limits spikes in blood sugar following a meal. Not only that, there's the "second meal effect": lentils have been shown to reduce blood glucose and food intake not just within the same meal but at the next meal, four hours later.[3] Lentils are also rich in lignins and other antioxidant compounds that have anti-cancer and anti-diabetic effects.[4]

Lentils and soybeans have more protein than almost any other plant food. Lentils are also a good source of iron for those eating plant-rich diets. Their plant proteins and other supportive nutrients also protect against muscle and bone loss with aging. They should be in everybody's diet.

DID YOU KNOW...?

Lentils need no pre-soaking, and cook much more quickly than other dried legumes.

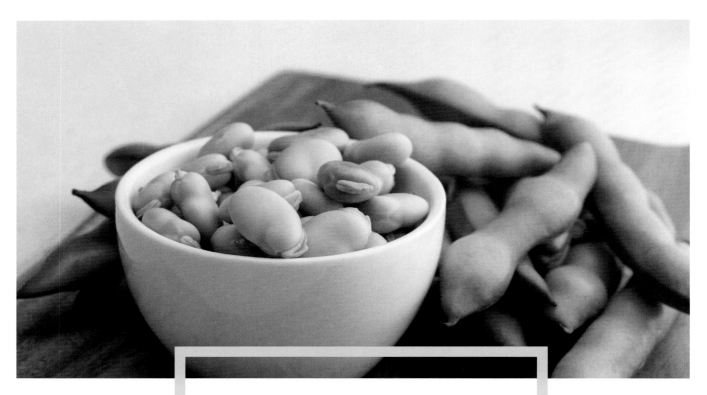

LIMA BEANS

Lima beans are so entrenched in Peruvian culture that they appear on the pottery of the Moche people, who inhabited northern Peru from 1 A.D. to the 8th century, and they are named after Lima, the capital of Peru. Lima Beans have more nicknames than any other bean: butter bean, Rangoon bean, Burma bean, Madagascar bean, and chad bean.

WHAT MAKES THEM SO SPECIAL?

Like most legumes, lima beans are a very good source of fiber, which helps reduce cholesterol levels, prevent colorectal cancers and prevent blood sugar levels from rising too rapidly after a meal.[1-3] These creamy, buttery flavored beans are not only low glycemic, but they also are an excellent source of molybdenum, an integral component of the enzyme sulfite oxidase, which is responsible for detoxifying sulfites. Lima beans supply loads of other minerals, too, and are an excellent source of magnesium, iron and folate – one cup of these pale green beans supplies about 25 percent of our iron requirements and two-thirds of our daily folate requirement. They are also rich in protein.

DID YOU KNOW?...

Lima beans are one of the main ingredients in succotash, a dish popular in the Southern U.S. You may have heard of it in your childhood: Looney Toons' cartoon cat Sylvester was famous for saying "Sufferin' succotash!"

MANGO

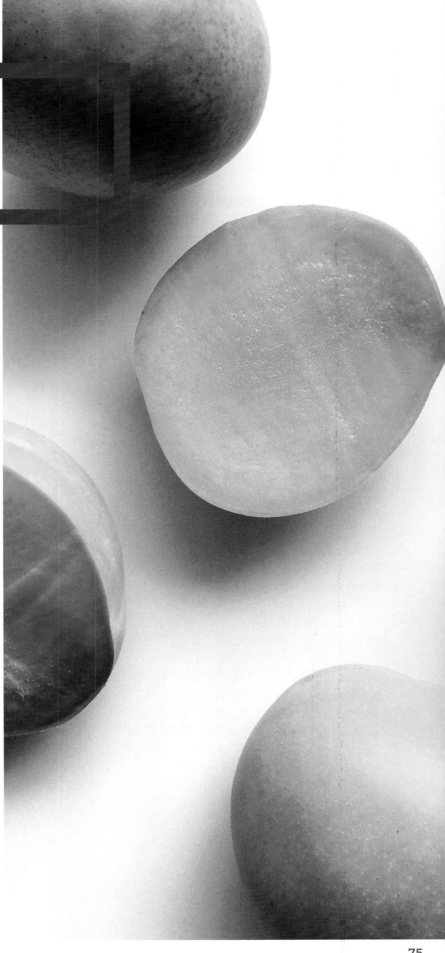

Mango is one of the most popular fruits in the world – it is the national fruit of India, Pakistan, and the Philippines. It is also the national tree of Bangladesh. There are many different varieties, all with their own distinct sweetness.

WHAT MAKES IT SO SPECIAL?

Mangoes contain an abundance of vitamins, carotenoids, fiber, and phytochemicals to help assure your good health.[1] In a study on humans, supplementation with mango powder every day for 12 weeks improved fasting blood glucose.[2] Research in cultured colon cancer cells suggests that mango phytochemicals may also have anti-cancer actions. Researchers treated the cells with extracts from common varieties of mangoes and found that growth of the cancerous cells was inhibited.[3]

MELONS

HONEYDEW

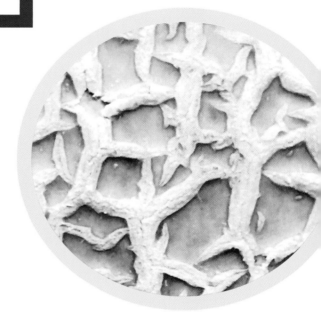

What Americans call a honeydew melon is known outside the U.S. as a White Antibes or Bailan melon. This variety was first cultivated centuries ago in southern France and Algeria.

WHAT MAKES IT SO SPECIAL?
The high water content of melons makes them an important food for those exercising in warm weather. Honeydew melons contain vitamin C and a variety of B vitamins, plus potassium and dietary fiber. One cup of honeydew melon supplies more than half of the body's daily requirement for vitamin C, an important antioxidant that helps to support immune function.

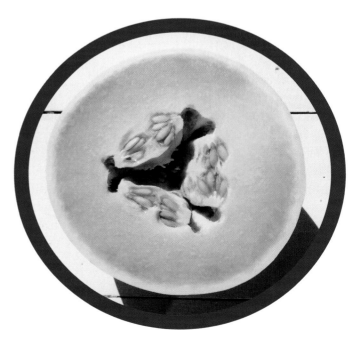

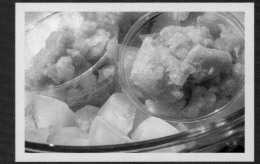

CANTALOUPE SLUSH
SERVES: 3

INGREDIENTS

1 cantaloupe, rind removed and seeded, and cut into pieces
2 cups ice
6 regular or 3 medjool dates, pitted

INSTRUCTIONS

1. Blend the ingredients together in a high-powered blender until smooth.

Variation: Use honeydew, peaches or nectarines instead of cantaloupe.

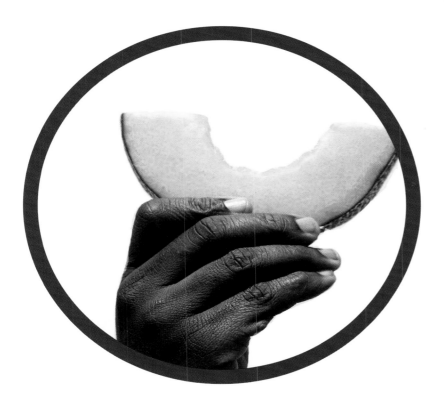

CANTALOUPE

The origin of the name "cantaloupe" is not known with certainty, but one theory is that the melons were given to Pope Paul II by Armenian envoys in the 15th century. The pope became very fond of the fruit and named it after Cantalupo di Sabina, the location of a papal estate, not far from Rome.

WHAT MAKES IT SO SPECIAL?

One cup of diced cantaloupe provides enough beta-carotene to meet the day's vitamin A recommendations, as well as a day's worth of vitamin C. Higher levels of carotenoids in the blood, including beta-carotene, are linked to greater telomere length of white blood cells. Telomeres give an indication of one's "biological age," with longer telomeres corresponding to younger biological age. Researchers think that carotenoids may protect telomeres from oxidative damage, potentially protecting against aging and chronic diseases.[1]

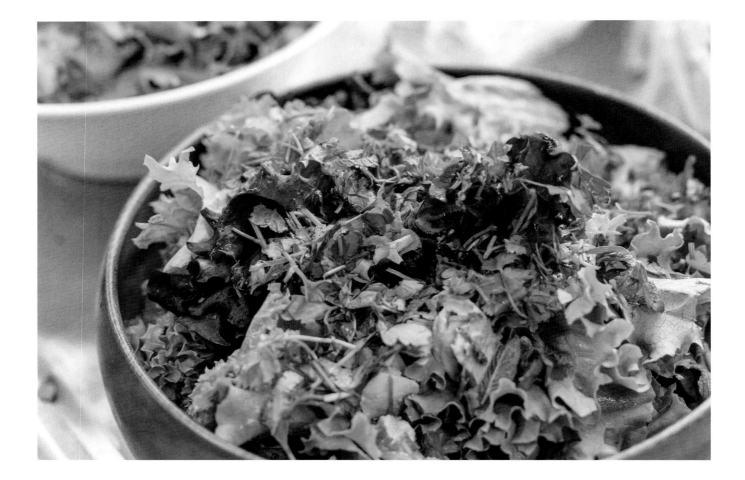

MIXED BABY GREENS

Packaged mixed greens are a convenient and quick way to make a salad and get a variety of raw vegetables.

WHAT MAKES THEM SO SPECIAL?

Eating a large salad at lunch and dinner is an excellent strategy for weight loss. Studies have found that women who were given salads either as a first course or as part of their main course consumed fewer calories from the whole meal. An important piece of this finding: the larger the salad, the better. [1,2] Eating salad greens regularly is also linked to a reduced risk of cardiovascular disease and cancer. For example, a two-cup serving of salad greens daily was associated with a 57 percent reduction in risk of stomach cancer.[3-5]

DID YOU KNOW...?

Caesar salad was not named after Julius Caesar. It was named after Caesar Cardini, the chef who invented it in 1924 at his restaurant in Tijuana.

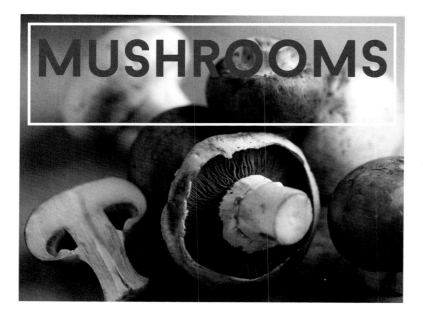

MUSHROOMS

Mushrooms are used in the culinary world as vegetables, but they are actually part of the fungi kingdom, which is completely separate from the plant kingdom. In ancient times, Egyptians and Asians used mushrooms to produce longevity tonics. Even Otzi the Iceman, the 5,300-year-old frozen mummy found in Europe in 1991, was carrying dried mushrooms with him when he died.

WHAT MAKES THEM SO SPECIAL?

Although they don't always get the respect they deserve, mushrooms are a superfood. Mushrooms are known for their unique polysaccharides, called beta-glucans, which have immune-boosting effects, thought to protect against infections and cancers.[1, 2] Other mushroom components interfere with estrogen production, which is likely why frequent consumption of mushrooms (approximately one button mushroom per day) has been linked to a 64 percent decrease in the risk of breast cancer.[3, 4] Mushroom phytochemicals also have anti-inflammatory effects that could help prevent cardiovascular disease.[5, 6] In addition, the fiber and potassium content of mushrooms all contribute to healthy blood pressure levels and good cardiovascular health. Mushrooms are rich in the B vitamins niacin and riboflavin, plus in the minerals potassium, iron, copper, and selenium.

DID YOU KNOW...?

Only eat mushrooms cooked. Common mushrooms (like white and Portobello) contain a potentially carcinogenic substance called agaritine, which is significantly reduced when mushrooms are heated.[7]

CREAMY MUSHROOM SOUP
SERVES: 4

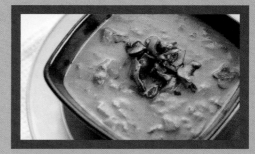

INGREDIENTS

20 ounces mushrooms, sliced
1 cup carrot juice
2 cups no-salt-added or low-sodium vegetable broth
1 large sweet onion
2 small carrots, sliced
2 tablespoons Dr.Fuhrman's Vegizest or other no-salt seasoning blend, adjusted to taste
1 1/2 teaspoons Bragg Liquid Aminos
4 cloves garlic, pressed
1 tablespoon fresh cilantro, or more to taste
1 cup walnuts
2 cups unsweetened soy, hemp or almond milk
1/4 teaspoon black pepper, or to taste

INSTRUCTIONS

1. Combine all ingredients except cilantro, walnuts, non-dairy milk and black pepper in a large pot. Cook about 25 minutes until carrots and mushrooms are tender.

2. Remove from heat and stir in fresh cilantro.

3. Pour 3/4 of the soup in a high-powered blender with the walnuts and non-dairy milk. Blend until smooth.

4. Pour mixture back into pot and stir.

5. Season with black pepper.

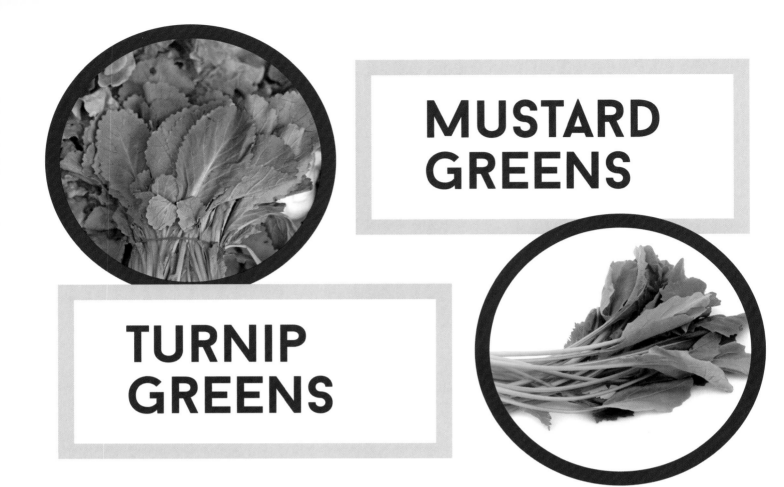

MUSTARD GREENS

TURNIP GREENS

Mustard greens and turnip greens have more in common than their sharp, peppery flavor. Both are leafy green cruciferous vegetables, both are staples of Southern cooking in the U.S., and both can be eaten raw or cooked (with cooking mellowing their flavors). Both plants also provide two distinct foods: mustard plants produce edible leaves, and also yellow flowers that contain mustard seeds, which are ground and used as a spice. Turnip plants produce edible greens, plus the more commonly-used white and purple turnip root. The two vegetables are members of the cabbage family, which also includes cauliflower, collards and broccoli.

WHAT MAKES THEM SO SPECIAL?

Both mustard greens and turnip greens have such a rich diversity of protective micronutrients and phytochemicals, that I put these greens, along with kale, watercress and arugula, at the apex of the Nutritarian Diet. They are the most powerful, disease-protecting, life-span enhancing foods on the planet. Mustard greens and turnip greens are anti-cancer superfoods, rich in many glucosinolates that convert into powerful disease-fighting compounds called isothiocyanates (ITCs).[1] These greens work great in soup recipes, but make sure to blend or chop finely when raw, before adding to the soup, to maximize the production of cancer-fighting ITCs. They are high in many different carotenoids, protecting against free radicals and LDL oxidation.[2] Mustard and turnip greens also protect our skin against damaging UV rays.[3,4] They contain the carotenoids lutein and zeaxanthin, which are important for eye health and protect against Age-related Macular Degeneration (AMD). They help protect the retina from damage and improve several aspects of visual performance.[5]

DID YOU KNOW...?

Both mustard and turnip greens are sweeter when harvested after a winter frost. The cold temperatures cause the vegetables to produce more sugar.

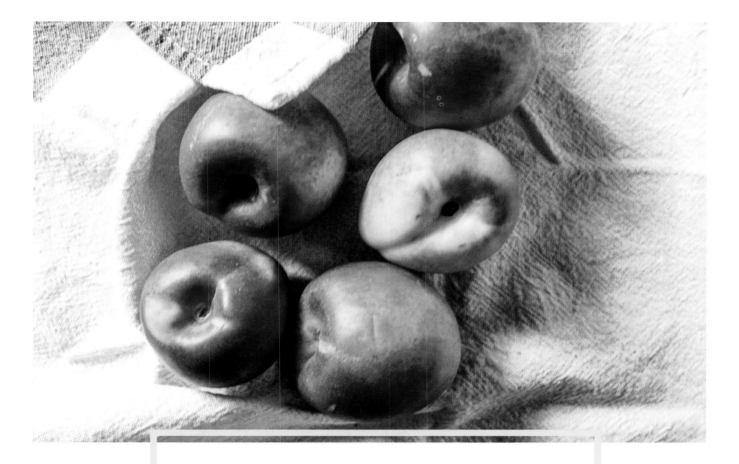

NECTARINES

Nectarines are actually peaches without the fuzzy skin. They first arose on naturally mutated branches on peach trees, which are native to China. By 1630, six different varieties of nectarines were being grown in England. This indicates that the "fuzz-less" peach had been selected by horticulturists, not only for its lack of fuzz, but also for characteristics such as tree vigor, fruit color and flavor.

WHAT MAKES THEM SO SPECIAL?

Eating nectarines and other stone fruit (fruit with flesh or pulp enclosing a stone, such as peach, apricot, plum and cherry) may benefit our cardiovascular health. This is due to the presence of heart-friendly antioxidants called proanthocyanidins, which are the most abundant antioxidant compounds in nectarines.[1-3] In the colon, proanthocyanidins act as prebiotics, promoting the growth of beneficial bacteria.[4] Proanthocyanidins also have anti-inflammatory, anti-proliferative, anti-angiogenic effects that help protect against cancer.[5] Don't try to eat the pits or seeds of nectarines or other stone fruits – the seeds look like almonds, but contain small amounts of cyanogens which, on ingestion, may get metabolized to cyanide. Although rare, excess ingestion of these pits may result in cyanide poisoning.

DID YOU KNOW...?

The name "nectarine" comes from the word "nectar," which is considered the sweet food of the gods.

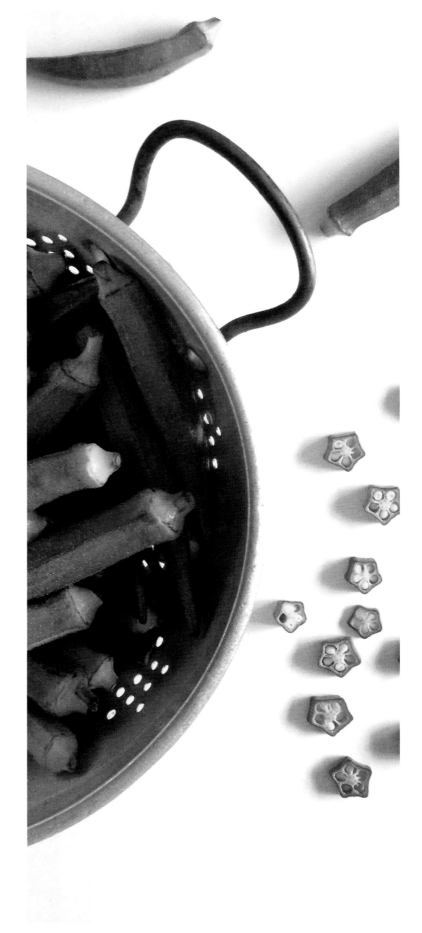OKRA

Okra consists of a pod with many seeds, and it is delicious to eat raw if the pods are small and still tender. It's a wonderful vegetable to grow at home. Okra is at its most tender, crisp and nutritious when it is fresh from the garden – it's great added to a salad or enjoyed with a dip. Okra seeds can be dried, toasted, and ground, to be used as a caffeine-free substitute for coffee. Frozen okra is a great addition to soups and other dishes. In the southern U.S., okra is a key ingredient in gumbo, which is a type of stew. The viscous fiber of the okra seeds gives the vegetable its characteristic "sliminess" when sliced and because of this, it is used to thicken the gumbo.

WHAT MAKES IT SO SPECIAL?

Like all greens, okra has hundreds of immune-boosting phytochemicals, but is also rich in protein and viscous fiber, which is especially helpful for those with diabetes or high cholesterol.[1] Okra is especially helpful when you want to lose weight, as it is satisfying and filling, yet low in calories. Big plus: it has the ability to hold fluid in the digestive tract, softening stools.

DID YOU KNOW...?

When picking okra out of the garden or from the market, remember to choose the smallest pods. Cut okra into pieces or cook the pods whole (just remove the stems). They blend nicely into many cooked dishes and combine especially well when a bit of acid flavoring, such as tomato, lemon juice or vinegar, is used while cooking.

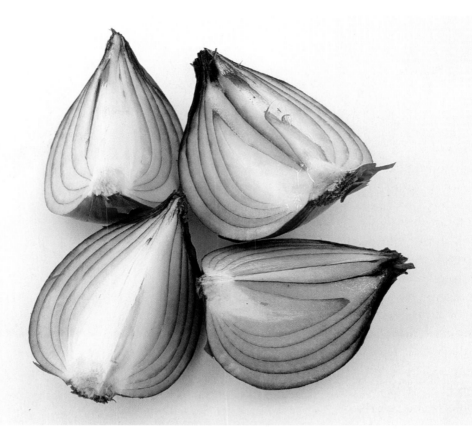

ONIONS

Little is known about the history of onions. Some archaeologists and researchers believe that this pungent vegetable is native to central Asia; others pinpoint its origins in Iran and West Pakistan. Since onions grew wild in various regions, it is presumed our ancestors discovered and started eating them very early – long before farming or even writing was invented. Very likely, onions were a staple in the prehistoric diet.

WHAT MAKES THEM SO SPECIAL?

Onions have beneficial effects on the cardiovascular and immune systems. Epidemiological studies have indicated that increased consumption of onions and other foods in the Allium family, like scallions and garlic, are also associated with a lower risk of gastric and prostate cancers.[1] Red onions contain at least 25 different flavonoid antioxidant anthocyanins, which have anti-inflammatory effects, and all onions contain high concentrations of quercetin, which slows tumor development, suppresses the growth and proliferation and induces cell death of colon cancer cells.[2-6] When preparing, be sure to chop or crush the onion finely before heating to release more of its helpful anti-cancer organosulfur compounds. These compounds prevent the development of cancers by detoxifying carcinogens, halting cancer cell growth, and blocking angiogenesis (blood vessel formation).[7] As part of my anti-cancer protocol, I strongly recommend eating some raw onion or scallion every day.

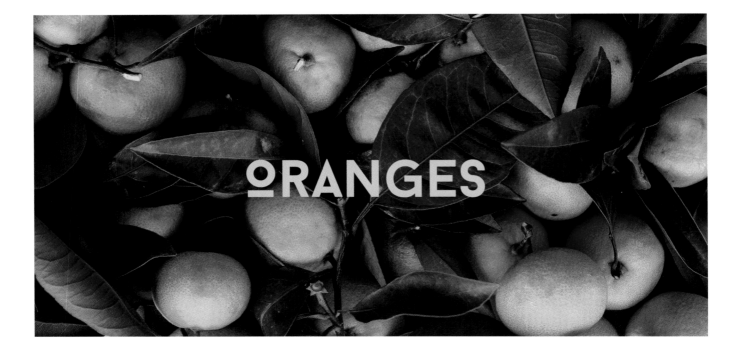

ORANGES

Although oranges first appeared in ancient text writings in 2200 B.C. and are believed to be native to tropical areas of Asia, we can most likely thank Ponce de Leon for bringing them to Florida in 1493.

WHAT MAKES THEM SO SPECIAL?

Oranges are a good source of fiber, thiamin and folate, with one fruit containing more than the daily recommended amount of vitamin C.

Vitamin C is also an important nutrient for the immune system and for fighting infection.

In addition to vitamins, oranges contain flavanones, especially hesperetin, which is known to lower cholesterol. Flavanones also help keep blood pressure down.[1]

PAPAYA

Although different parts of the world cultivate their own varieties, the two major types of papaya in the U.S. are Mexican and Hawaiian. Mexican papayas are fairly large fruits and can reach weights up to 10 pounds. The Hawaiian papayas are much smaller.

WHAT MAKES IT SO SPECIAL?

When researchers tested papaya against other carotenoid sources (carrots and tomatoes), they found that beta-carotene and lycopene from papaya were better absorbed than from raw carrots or tomatoes.[1] Papaya has been shown in studies to have antioxidant and anti-inflammatory properties.[2-4] The seeds of the papaya are edible, but have a peppery taste, and are sometimes ground and used as a seasoning. Papayas are extremely perishable; once ripe, they have a short shelf life. Enjoy them soon after they become yellow, and store them in the fridge as soon as they ripen.

DID YOU KNOW..?

Explorer Christopher Columbus is said to have called called papaya "the fruit of the angels."

PARSNIPS

Parsnips were used as a sweetening agent for foods before cane sugar became a major import in North America in the 17th century. In the past, wild parsnips were even used in herbal medicine and as an aphrodisiac.

WHAT MAKES THEM SO SPECIAL?

They can be eaten raw or cooked and add a great flavor to soups and stews. Parsnips have a high fiber content, half of which is soluble fiber, the variety that helps reduce cholesterol levels.[1] Furthermore, a high-fiber diet is a key component of great health, facilitating healthy movement of food through the digestive tract, feeding the microbiome, and contributing to a reduced risk of heart disease, diabetes, and cancer.[2]

DID YOU KNOW..?

Parsnips are available all year round. Because they gain a sweetness that comes from being frozen in the ground, the winter ones are often the tastiest. Smaller parsnips are generally sweeter and less woody than larger ones. Look for parsnips that are heavy for their size; they will be sweeter as well.

PEACHES

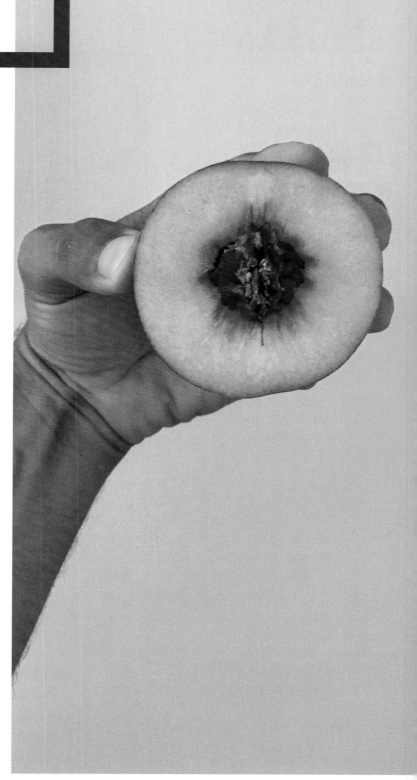

Amazingly, well before modern man emerged, peaches made their appearance. In 2015, scientists found eight fossilized peach endocarps (pits) in southwest China thought to be more than 2.5 million years old. Despite their age, these fossils appeared almost identical to the peach pits of today, though somewhat smaller.

WHAT MAKES THEM SO SPECIAL?

Peaches have great health benefits, from helping to kill cancer cells to making you look better. Breast cancer cells, even aggressive ones, died after being treated with peach and plum extracts in the lab – most importantly, without harming normal cells. It was determined that two specific phytochemicals, chlorogenic acid and neochlorogenic acid, were responsible for the cancer-fighting effects.[1] Though they are very common in fruits, stone fruits such as peaches and plums are especially rich in these phytochemicals.

DID YOU KNOW...?

You can easily remove the skin from peaches that are not organic by dipping them in boiling water for 30 seconds and then transferring them immediately to an ice bath. (Of course, do not remove the skins of organic peaches.) If you have a peach tree, you can purchase an expandable picking wand with a basket on the end to reach up to the top of the tree.

POMEGRANATE POACHED PEARS
SERVES: 6

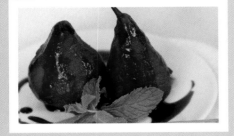

INGREDIENTS
6 medium pears
2 cups pomegranate juice
1 whole cinnamon stick
6 whole cloves
2 tablespoons Goji berries

FOR THE CHOCOLATE SAUCE
1 cup frozen blueberries
1 1/2 cups unsweetened soy, hemp or almond milk
1 cup pitted dates
2/3 cup raw macadamia nuts
1 tablespoon unsweetened natural cocoa powder, or more for a darker, stronger sauce
1/2 teaspoon vanilla extract
1 teaspoon turmeric

FOR THE RASPBERRY SAUCE
1 1/2 cup frozen red raspberries, thawed

INSTRUCTIONS
1. Slice a little off the bottom of each peeled pear. In a large sauce pan, place pears standing up.

2. Pour in pomegranate juice. Add cinnamon, cloves and Goji berries. Gently simmer, covered, for about 20 minutes until pears are tender.

3. Remove pears and refrigerate until ready to serve. Reduce liquid until it becomes a syrup.

4. Place blueberries, non-dairy milk, dates, macadamia nuts, cocoa powder, vanilla and turmeric in blender. Blend until very smooth and creamy. Add more milk if needed.

5. Place defrosted raspberries in a blender and blend until smooth. Mix in syrup. Place a generous dollop of chocolate sauce on dessert plate. Place pear on chocolate and drizzle raspberry sauce over pear.

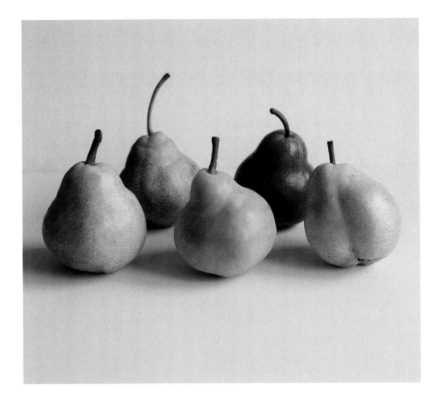

PEARS

One of the oldest fruit crops, pears have been cultivated for more than 3,000 years. Pear trees are thought to have originated 55 to 65 million years ago in southwestern China.

WHAT MAKES THEM SO SPECIAL?
Pears provide potassium, fiber, and vitamin C. Don't peel pears when eating them raw– most of the vitamin C and other antioxidant phytochemicals are in the skin. These phytonutrients include antioxidant, anti-inflammatory flavonoids, one called quercetin in particular.[1] In 2011, a large study on fruit and vegetable consumption and stroke risk divided up the foods by color. White fruits and vegetables – a group composed of more than half apples and pears – had a strong relationship with a lower risk of stroke.[2] The scientists think that the high fiber and quercetin content of apples and pears may be responsible, as both of these components have blood pressure-lowering properties.[3,4]

DID YOU KNOW...?
Pears are a part of the rose family.

PEAS

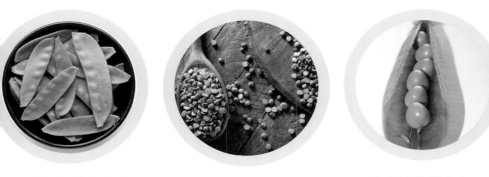

SNOW   SPLIT   GREEN

Peas are rich in fiber and, like beans, are a healthful and low-glycemic starch source. Shelled peas are green because they are harvested when not mature; if allowed to fully ripen, they would be yellow. Split peas are green or yellow peas grown specifically to be dried. The pods of both the sugar snap and snow pea varieties are edible.

WHAT MAKES THEM SO SPECIAL?
No matter the variety, peas are high in both vitamin C and vitamin K. One of the phytonutrients in peas, a phytoestrogen called coumestrol, has been recognized for its ability to offer protection from stomach cancer. A Mexico City-based study indicated that the daily consumption of green peas lowers the risk of stomach cancer.[1] Coumestrol has demonstrated growth inhibitory effects in breast cancer cells, and higher coumestrol intake was associated with a lower risk of hormone receptor negative breast cancers. [2, 3] Split peas contain isoflavones – daidzein in particular.[4] These are the same phytochemicals found in soybeans that are thought to help decrease the risk of certain types of cancers, especially breast cancer and prostate cancer.[5-8] Peas are rich in fiber and resistant starch; eating these legumes regularly helps to keep cholesterol and blood sugar down, and prevent heart disease and colon cancer.[9-13]

DID YOU KNOW...?
Peas are one of the few vegetables that are almost better when purchased frozen. That's because the longer peas sit after being picked, the more their sugars turn into starch. They are also a great food to grow because you can eat the peas and its leaves, which are delicious in a salad.

HERBED SPLIT PEA SOUP
SERVES: 4

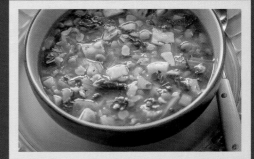

INGREDIENTS
1 3/4 cups dried split peas
4 cups low-sodium or no-salt-added vegetable broth
3 cups water
2 cloves garlic, minced
1/4 teaspoon dried sage
1 teaspoon dried basil
1/2 teaspoon dried thyme
1 tablespoon salt-free poultry seasoning
1/2 cup diced onion
1/2 cup sliced carrots
1/2 cup sliced celery
1/2 cup bite-sized pieces white or sweet potato
4 packed cups kale or spinach

INSTRUCTIONS
1. Combine split peas, broth, water, garlic, sage, basil, thyme, and poultry seasoning. Cover and simmer for 30 minutes, stirring occasionally so the split peas don't stick to the bottom of the pot.

2. Add onions, carrots, celery, and potatoes. Cover and simmer for another 30 minutes or until vegetables are tender. If using kale, add during the last 15 minutes of cooking time; If using spinach, add at the end of the cooking time and heat until just wilted.

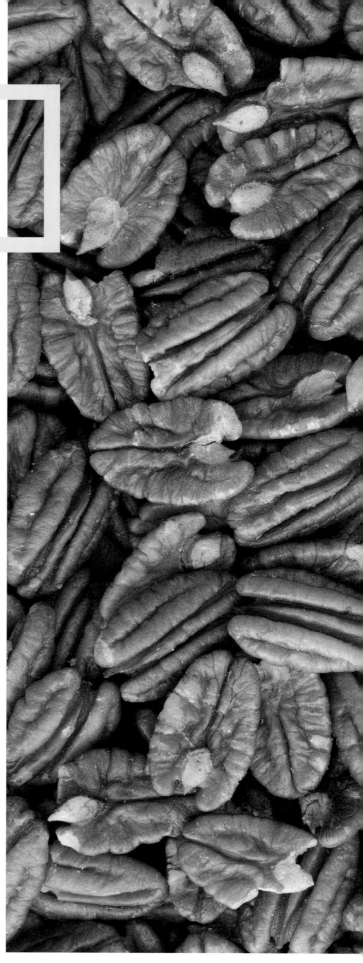

PECANS

Early Native Americans ate wild pecans and named them "pacane," an Algonquin word which means "nuts requiring a stone to crack." Pecans are a major agricultural product in many of the southern states – it is estimated that the U.S. produces 75 percent of the world's pecans.

WHAT MAKES THEM SO SPECIAL?

In addition to their distinctive flavor and texture, pecans are rich in fiber, vitamin E and zinc. The nuts are especially rich in antioxidant phytochemicals; pecans and walnuts rank highest in total phenols (a large class of phytochemicals).[1] Study participants who added pecans to the diet, as you might then expect, increased the total antioxidant capacity of their blood and reduced markers of oxidation of LDL cholesterol.[2] Similar to other nuts, pecans are a health-promoting, high-fat whole food that helps keep LDL cholesterol levels down.[3] Nut consumption overall is linked to a longer life and a reduced risk of both cancer and cardiovascular disease.[4, 5]

DID YOU KNOW...?

What's the correct pronunciation of pecan? There isn't one, according to the Merriam-Webster dictionary, which lists three accepted pronunciations for the word.

PEPPERS
(BELL)

The most common colors of bell peppers (also called sweet peppers) are green, yellow, orange and red, though you can also find brown, white, lavender, and purple varieties. Green peppers are actually unripe peppers and, as a result, are less sweet than the more colorful varieties. Red bell peppers are the sweetest.

WHAT MAKES THEM SO SPECIAL?

Although all bell peppers are high in vitamin C, red peppers have the highest amount; a large one can contain 300 percent of your daily requirement. Red peppers also contain several phytochemicals and carotenoids including lycopene, an antioxidant with powerful anti-cancer effects. The carotenoids capsanthin and capsorubin, found only in red peppers, were found to protect skin cells against UV-induced DNA damage.[1] In fact, capsanthin gives red peppers their color.[2] Luteolin is a flavonoid abundant in green peppers, which has anti-inflammatory, antioxidant, and anti-cancer properties.[3] Luteolin has been shown to block the growth of human colon cancer cells by interfering with growth signals from insulin-like growth factor 1 (IGF-1), a hormone that in excess promotes cancer and aging.[4, 5]

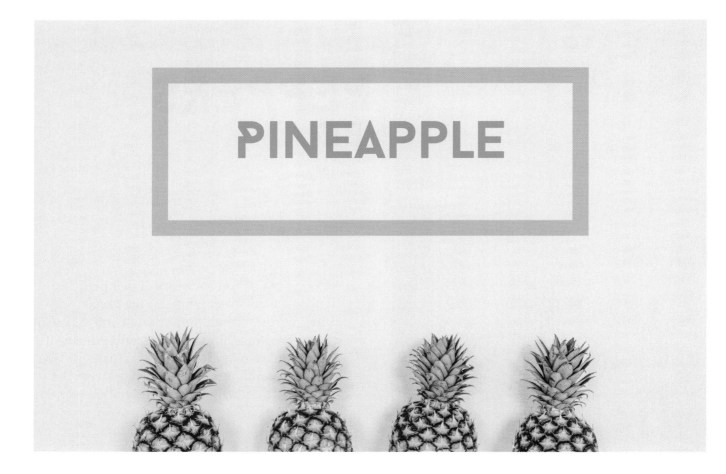

PINEAPPLE

Despite what many people believe, pineapple is not native to Hawaii, but rather to South America. It is believed the fruit's name was inspired by its resemblance to a pine cone.

WHAT MAKES IT SO SPECIAL?

Bromelain is an enzyme extracted from the flesh and stem of the pineapple plant.[1] It has many known benefits. It is rich in polyphenols such as ferulic and coumaric acid which have anti-inflammatory and a variety of anti-cancer effects, and pineapple fiber also inhibits cancer cell proliferation.[1-3] Pineapple extract in vitro protects DNA against carcinogens.[4] One cup of pineapple provides 75 percent of the daily recommended amount of the mineral manganese. This mineral is essential for developing strong bones and connective tissue, and for the workings of the body's antioxidant system.[5]

DID YOU KNOW...?

Pineapple does not continue to sweeten after it is harvested, so it's important to choose one with a yellow-gold tinge that has already ripened while still on the plant. The bottom end of the pineapple is the sweetest and most ripe; for the best flavor, choose a pineapple whose yellow color reaches as far to the top end of the fruit as possible, and whose leaves are bright green. Deterioration is indicated by a wrinkling in the skin and browning of the leaves.

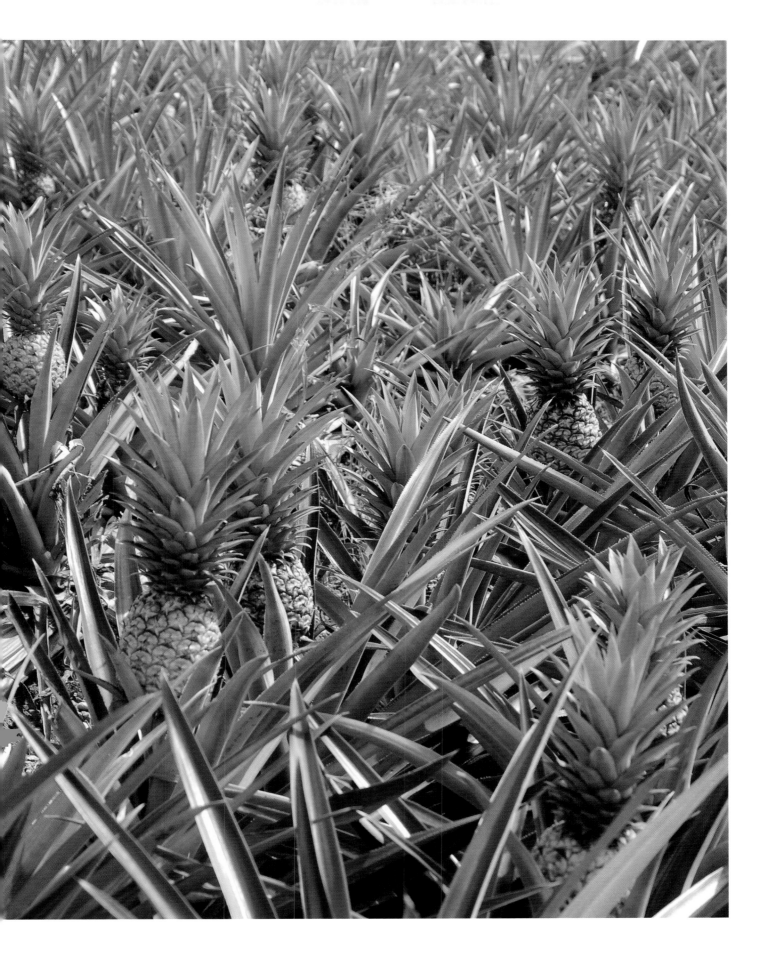

DID YOU KNOW...?

Mediterranean or Stone Pine Nuts (Pinus pinea) are considered the finest as they grow on trees that are many hundreds of years old and their high protein content makes them a great food for athletes. They are native to Italy, Spain, and Portugal. Their flavor is complex, yet lighter and more delicate than the more common, widely available Chinese, Korean or Mexican pine nuts. You can tell them apart by the shape: most pine nuts are cone-shaped, whereas Mediterranean pine nuts are longer and symmetrical at both ends.

PINE NUTS

ASPARAGUS WITH PINE NUT VINAGRETTE
SERVES: 4

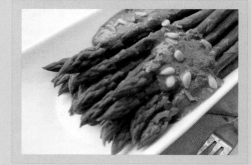

Although the name should give it away, many people don't realize that pine nuts actually come from pine cones. Pine nuts can take anywhere from 18 months to 3 years to mature. To harvest, the cones are dried in a burlap bag in the sun for weeks. The cones are then smashed, and the seeds are separated by hand from the cone fragments. This is a time-consuming process, and plays a part in the high cost of pine nuts. There are hundreds of varieties of pine nuts and it has been an important food throughout human history in many regions of the world.

WHAT MAKES THEM SO SPECIAL?

Pine nuts provide significant amounts of protein, vitamin E and minerals magnesium, zinc, phosphorus, copper, and manganese. Pinolenic acid, a fatty acid derived from pine nuts, was found to reduce appetite in women by increasing secretion of satiety hormones.[1,2] Mediterranean pine nuts have almost 30 percent protein – double the protein content compared to Chinese pine nuts – and are one of the richest whole food sources of plant sterols.[3,4] Plant sterols have a similar structure to cholesterol, and are able to inhibit the re-absorption of cholesterol in the digestive system, leading to excretion of the cholesterol and helping to maintain favorable blood cholesterol levels.[5] In addition to their cholesterol-lowering properties, higher plant sterol intake has been linked to a lower risk of several common cancers.[6-10]

INGREDIENTS
2 pounds asparagus, tough ends removed
1/2 cup water
1/4 cup balsamic vinegar
1/4 cup walnuts
1/2 cup raisins
1 teaspoon Dijon mustard
1 clove garlic, chopped
2 tablespoons chopped red onion
1 red bell pepper, roasted and sliced
2 tablespoons pine nuts, lightly toasted
1 tablespoon chopped fresh tarragon

INSTRUCTIONS
1. Steam asparagus for 8-10 minutes or until crisp-tender.

2. Combine water, vinegar, walnuts, raisins, mustard, and garlic in a high-powered blender. Stir in red onion. Mix with asparagus just before serving. Add roasted red pepper.

3. Sprinkle with pine nuts and tarragon.

PISTACHIO AVOCADO GELATO

SERVES: 8

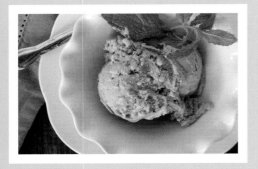

INGREDIENTS
3/4 cup unsalted shelled pistachios, divided
2 cups water
1/2 cup raw cashews
2/3 cup silken tofu
18 regular dates or 9 Medjool dates, pitted
1 cup frozen mango chunks
1 small or 1/2 large avocado
1 handful raw spinach
1/4 teaspoon almond extract

INSTRUCTIONS
1. Coarsely chop ¼ cup of the 3/4 cup raw pistachios and set aside to add later.

2. Blend the other 1/2 cup of pistachios along with remaining ingredients in a high-powered blender until smooth and creamy.

3. Stir in chopped pistachios.

4. Freeze in an ice cream maker or freezer.

PISTACHIO NUTS

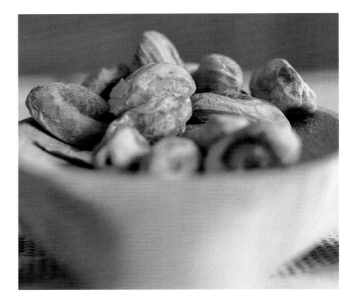

Both male and female pistachio trees are needed to bear fruit – the pollination is enabled by the wind, which carries the pollen from the male trees to the female ones. In China, pistachios are known as "the happy nut" because the open shells make it look like the nut is smiling.

WHAT MAKES THEM SO SPECIAL?
Pistachios have the highest plant sterol content of all nuts, which could be another reason they look so happy. Peanuts have a slightly higher amount, but aren't considered a true nut – they are a legume. Plant sterols are structurally similar to cholesterol, and help to lower cholesterol levels.[1] Pistachios reduce inflammation and oxidative stress as well.[2-4] In addition to antioxidants and plant sterols, pistachios are also rich in arginine, an amino acid that helps maintain healthy levels of blood pressure and blood flow.[4]

DID YOU KNOW...?
According to a small study done in 2011, men who consumed 100 grams of pistachios (just over 3 ounces) a day for 3 weeks improved their erectile function, blood flow, and cholesterol levels.[5] Who needs Viagra? Just eat some pistachios!

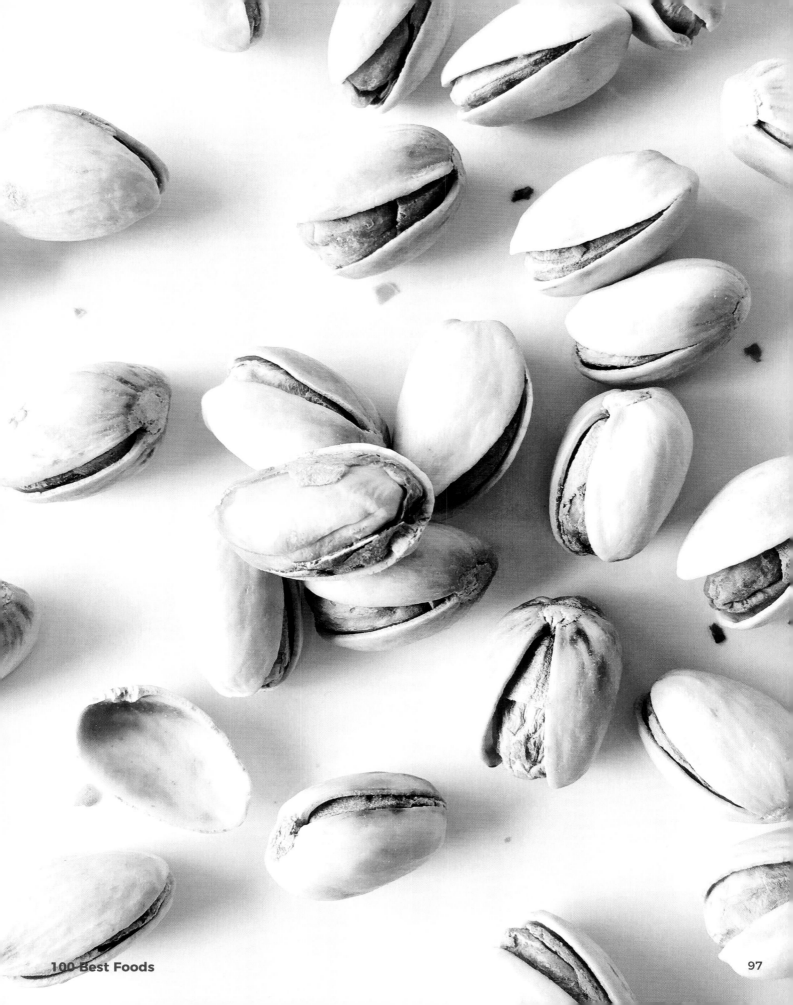

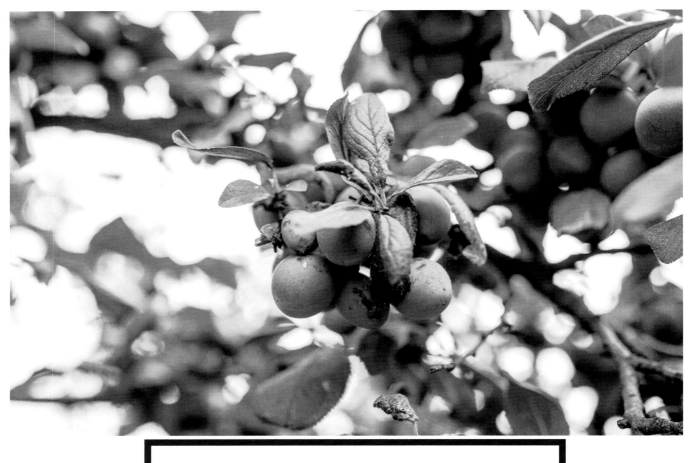

PLUMS

Plums are thought to have been one of the first fruits domesticated by humans. The remains of this delicious fruit have been found in Neolithic age archaeological sites along with olives, grapes and figs.

WHAT MAKES THEM SO SPECIAL?

Dried plums (prunes) are known for their ability to relieve constipation.[1] However, more recent research has revealed that plums may also have potent bone-building effects that help to prevent osteoporosis. Studies, primarily in postmenopausal women, have investigated biomarkers of bone health or bone density, many of which suggest that eating fresh or dried plums daily could be an effective strategy to preserve bone health.[2] Plums are rich in polyphenols – the most abundant are chlorogenic acid, neochlorogenic acid, and cryptochlorogenic acid – that help to counteract the oxidative stress and inflammation that is linked to bone loss. Plums also contain vitamin K and the minerals boron, copper, and potassium, which also have roles in bone health. [2]

DID YOU KNOW...?

Plum trees are grown on every continent except Antarctica.

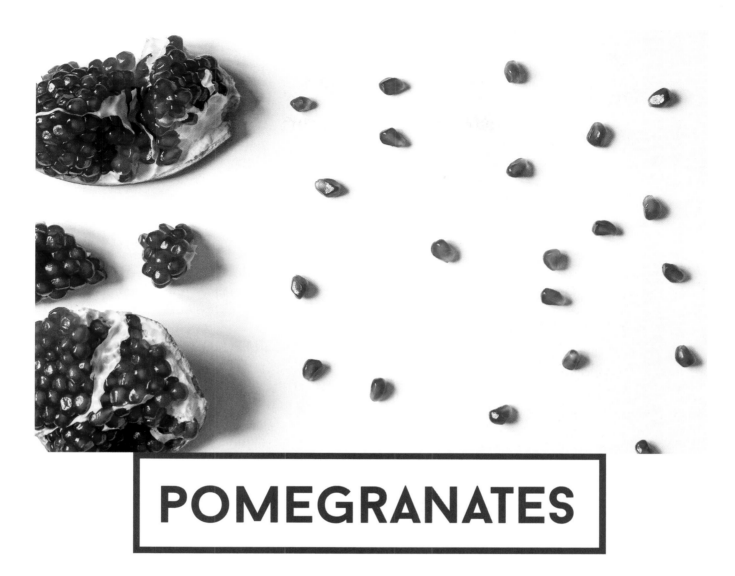

POMEGRANATES

For thousands of years, pomegranates have been used all over the world as medicine, thanks to their healing properties. More recently, pomegranates have been shown in laboratory tests to have antiviral, antibacterial and antioxidant properties.[1, 2]

WHAT MAKES THEM SO SPECIAL?

In the laboratory it was shown that extracts of the juice, rind and oil of pomegranates slowed down the reproduction of cancer cells, and also helped reduce the blood supply to tumors, thereby starving them and preventing them from growing.[3] Patients with prostate cancer who took pomegranate extract or pomegranate juice daily had slower PSA doubling time, which suggests that pomegranates could help to prevent recurrence of prostate cancer.[4, 5]

There have also been studies in humans, suggesting that pomegranate juice protects LDL cholesterol from oxidation,[2] and also improves blood pressure and shrinks coronary artery blockages.[6] Research also suggests that the fruit's potent antioxidant capacity provides protection against cognitive impairment.[7] It is best to eat the arils (seeds), rather than juice the pomegranate, to get more of its health benefits.

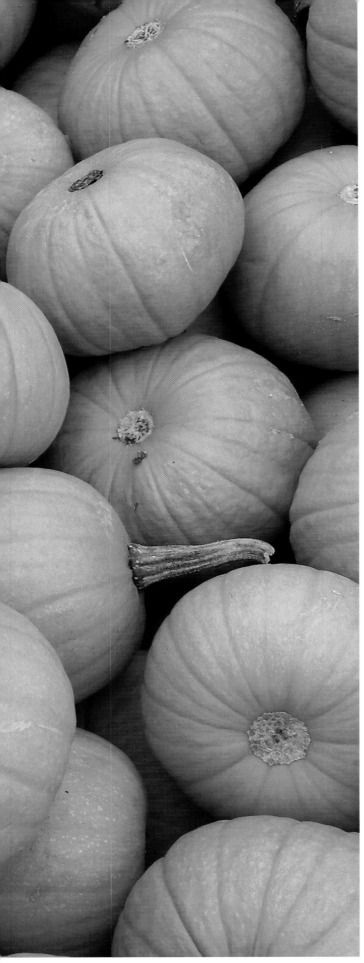

PUMPKIN

Pumpkins were part of the Native American diet centuries before the Pilgrims landed in 1620 and discovered their many uses. The indigenous people taught the settlers how to cultivate and use the versatile veggie: they'd eat them boiled, or roasted over an open fire; they also dried strips of pumpkin and wove them into mats. Native Americans considered pumpkins, beans and corn to be "the three sisters" – crops that support one another when planted together: Pumpkin leaves shade the roots of the corn; corn stalks support the bean vines; and bean roots supply nitrogen to the soil.

WHAT MAKES IT SO SPECIAL?

This orange-colored member of the squash family, associated with Halloween and the fall season, is loaded with nutrients. One cup of cubed pumpkin contains only 30 calories, and 17 percent of the daily requirement for vitamin C. Pumpkin is very rich in carotenoids, with enough beta-carotene, alpha-carotene, and beta-cryptoxanthin in one cup to supply more than double your daily vitamin A recommendation, plus lutein and zeaxanthin. Carotenoids are major antioxidant nutrients, and higher circulating carotenoid levels are linked to a longer life.[1-3] Vitamin A has been found to slow the decline of retinal function in those with retinitis pigmentosa, a degenerative eye disease that can lead to blindness. Pumpkin also provides significant amounts of vitamin C, vitamin E, and potassium. When buying a pumpkin, choose one that is firm and heavy for its size. And don't forget: In addition to its tasty flesh, those seeds inside the pumpkin are perfect for toasting and filled with nutrients – they're even one of my top 100 Best Foods!

DID YOU KNOW...?

The world's largest pumpkin, from Germany, was grown in 2016 and weighed 2,624 pounds. If you consider that the entire fruit is edible, including the pulp, seeds, skin and flowers; you can imagine how many people that can serve.

PUMPKIN SEEDS

Some people think the seed is the best part of the pumpkin. The seeds with white shells we find in our own pumpkins are different from the smaller green seeds, known as pepitas, that we find in stores. Pepitas come from a variety of pumpkin whose seeds don't have shells.

WHAT MAKES THEM SO SPECIAL?

Small, but mighty in essential nutrients, pumpkin seeds are a great source of minerals, especially iron, magnesium, zinc, copper, and manganese. Among plant foods, pumpkin seeds are the richest source of zinc. This makes them an especially helpful food for vegetarians and vegans, since zinc is more absorbable from animal foods than from plant foods. Among its many different functions in the body, zinc is essential for the proper functioning of many different types of immune cells.[1-5] Among nuts and seeds, pumpkin seeds are also uniquely high in vitamin K, less like a seed and more like a leafy green vegetable; pumpkin seeds provide 17 percent of the daily recommended intake of this vitamin in one ounce.

PUMPKIN PIE SMOOTHIE
SERVES: 2

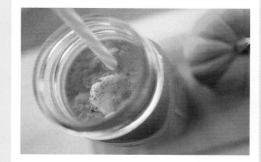

INGREDIENTS

1 cup unsweetened vanilla soy, hemp or almond milk
1 banana, peeled and frozen
2 medjool or 4 regular dates, pitted
1 cup pumpkin puree (see note)
2 cups spinach
2 cups romaine lettuce
2 ice cubes
1/4 teaspoon cinnamon
1/8 teaspoon ground nutmeg

INSTRUCTIONS

1. Place all ingredients in a high-powered blender.

2. Process on high until smooth and creamy.

Note: Use fresh pumpkin puree or pumpkin puree packed in a non-BPA container.

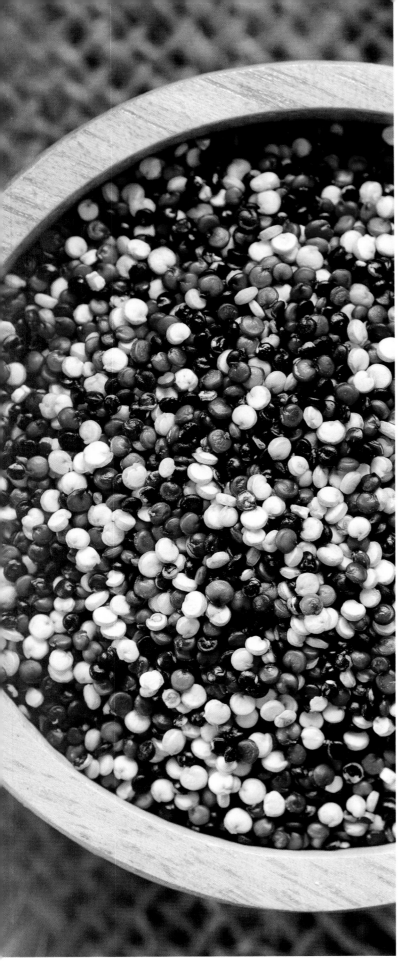

QUINOA

For 5,000 years quinoa has been above it all – and still is. Grown at 10,000 to 20,000 feet above sea level, quinoa is native to Peru and Bolivia, and is sometimes referred to as "the golden grain of the Andes." In fact, quinoa is botanically related to beets, chard and spinach.

WHAT MAKES IT SO SPECIAL?

One cup of quinoa provides 30 percent of your daily requirement for magnesium – a critical mineral for every cell in the body, important for bone health and favorable blood pressure.[1] In addition, quinoa is low-glycemic and nutrient-dense, providing fiber, iron, B vitamins, calcium, potassium, phosphorus, and vitamin E. It also contains antioxidant flavonoids such as betalains, which fight aging and protect against disease. Studies on adding quinoa to the diet have found reduced oxidative stress, cholesterol, and triglycerides.[2,3] Buy pre-washed quinoa varieties or rinse before cooking, because raw quinoa grains are naturally coated with saponins that are bitter and mildly toxic in large doses. When buying quinoa in bulk, filter it carefully before cooking – it can contain tiny rocks mixed with the grains.

100 Best Foods

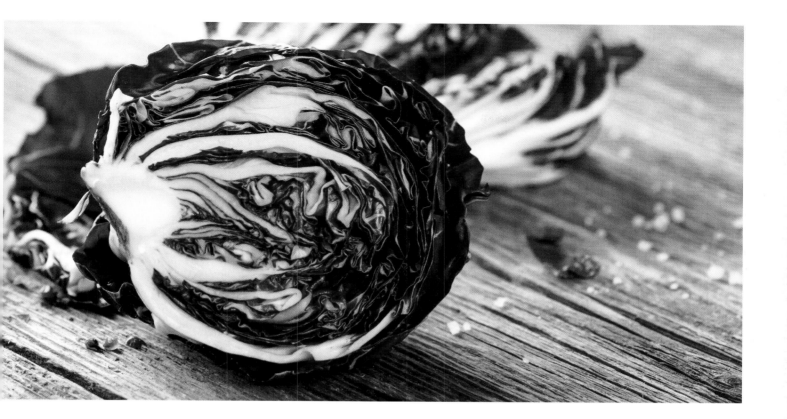

RADICCHIO

There are many different varieties of radicchio, with their names indicating the regions of northern Italy in which they are grown. The deep-red radicchio we see most often today, Rosso di Verona, was developed in the late 1800s using a technique called imbianchimento (whitening) to produce white veins in the dark red leaves. The technique involves withholding light for part of the plant's life.

WHAT MAKES IT SO SPECIAL?

A member of the chicory family, radicchio is rich in anthocyanins, a class of flavonoid antioxidants. Not all flavonoids are absorbed from foods, but those that aren't can reach the colon, where they have beneficial effects on those cells. Radicchio anthocyanins were shown to protect colon epithelial cells that had been exposed to oxidative stress.[1,2] Anthocyanins are also known for their cardioprotective effects. Radicchio's degree of bitterness depends on the variety; Treviso, Chioggia and Castelfranco are milder in flavor than the Verona variety.

DID YOU KNOW...?

This vibrant veggie did not make its way into many Western kitchens until restaurants started using it in 1977, when the New York Times food editor, Craig Claiborne, discovered it and wrote about it while on a trip to Italy.

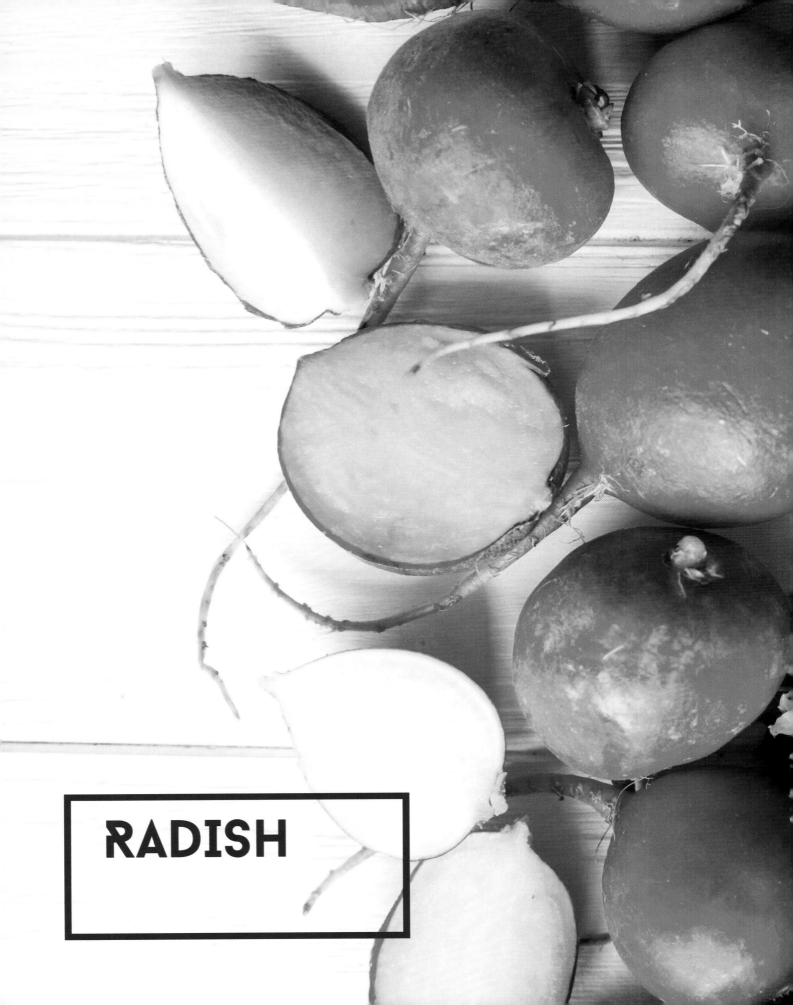

RADISH

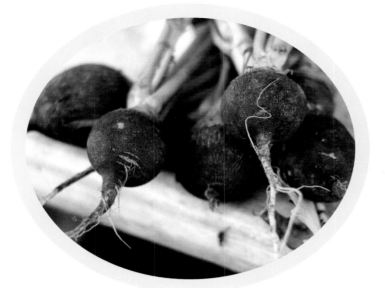

Radishes were so revered in ancient Greece that radish replicas were made of Gold. Oaxaca, Mexico celebrates The Night of Radishes (Noche de Rabanos) on December 23rd, when radishes are carved into shapes similar to the Halloween tradition of carving pumpkins.

WHAT MAKES IT SO SPECIAL?

Radishes are a great source of anthocyanins, a type of flavonoid, which provide numerous health benefits. Anthocyanins have been the subject of numerous medical studies, and have been positively linked to reducing the occurrence of cardiovascular disease. They also have displayed anti-inflammatory properties as well as anti-cancer properties, and are particularly protective against colon, kidney, intestinal, stomach, and oral cancers. The major isothiocyanate (ITC) found in radishes, sulforaphene (a phytochemical somewhat similar to sulforaphane in broccoli), has a major impact on the workings of cancerous cells, causing apoptosis (cell death), thereby preventing cancerous cells from reproducing.[1-3] Radish is another cruciferous vegetable that is best eaten raw, and adding it to salads is a major boon.

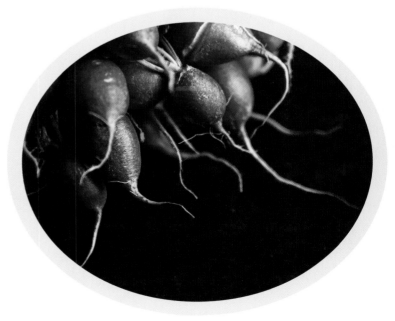

RASPBERRIES

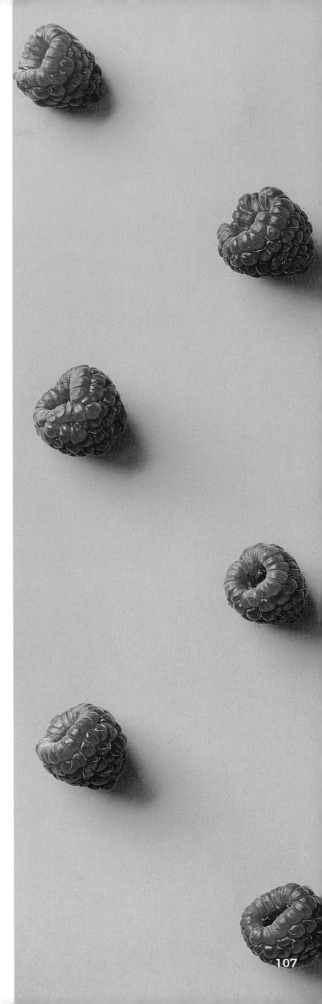

According to Greek mythology, raspberries were originally white, until Zeus' nursemaid, Ida, pricked her finger on one of the thorns, coloring the berries red. While there is historical evidence that the raspberry was valued for its sweetness, the leaves were also valuable, as they were used in medicinal preparations. The most common colors are red and black, but raspberries also come in shades of purple, orange and golden yellow.

WHAT MAKES THEM SO SPECIAL?

A raspberry is made up of many tiny bead-like fruits called "drupelets" clustered around a core. Each drupelet contains one seed, and a typical raspberry has 100 to 120 seeds. Red raspberries contain powerful antioxidants such as anthocyanins and ellagitannins, which have protective effects against heart disease, diabetes, and cancer. In vitro studies show red raspberry extract increases antioxidant enzyme activity within the cells, decreases the activity of pro-inflammatory substances, inhibits DNA damage, and slows the breakdown of starches by digestive enzymes.[1] Black raspberries have been used in exciting new studies on cancers and precancerous conditions. Black raspberry gel was applied to precancerous lesions in the mouth twice a day for 12 weeks; in the black raspberry group, on average the patients' lesions showed a reduction in size, whereas in the placebo group, lesions increased in size. The black raspberry group also experienced a reduction in histologic grade, meaning that the progression to cancer started to reverse.[2] Another clinical trial in patients with colorectal cancer reported a reduction in blood inflammatory markers, plus a reduction in proliferation and angiogenesis markers in the cancerous tissue after patients consumed freeze-dried black raspberry powder three times a day for three weeks.[3] All types of raspberries are longevity-promoting foods with a portfolio of health benefits.

DID YOU KNOW...?

Like watermelons, grapes and blueberries, raspberries do not continue to ripen after they are picked because they are non-climacteric fruit, which means they produce little or no ethylene gas.

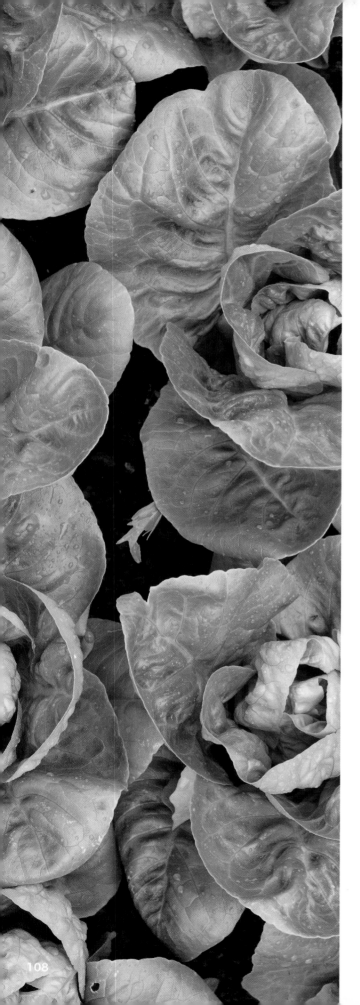

ROMAINE LETTUCE

Romaine is among the oldest of cultivated lettuces. Its 5,000 year history spans from a bitter weed to a food plant grown for its succulent leaves and oil-rich seeds.

WHAT MAKES IT SO SPECIAL?

Romaine supplies a wide range of vitamins, minerals and antioxidants, including beta-carotene, folate, and vitamin K. It is the most nutrient-rich and flavorful variety of lettuce. A 100 gram serving (3.5 ounces, or about 2 cups of shredded romaine) supplies 174 percent of your daily requirement for vitamin A via beta-carotene; 40 percent for vitamin C; and 34 percent for folate. The same amount of iceberg lettuce, by contrast, supplies only 10 percent of your daily vitamin A, and 7 percent for folate. Folate is a B vitamin that is especially important for pregnant women, because it helps prevent neural tube defects during fetal development. But that's not all – getting adequate folate is essential for protection against cancer. The safest way to get your folate is from foods, as supplemental folic acid has been linked to an increased risk of cancer in several studies.[1-3]

RUTABAGA

Rutabaga is a root vegetable that looks like its relative, the turnip. Smaller rutabagas tend to be sweeter than larger ones. Although this hardy vegetable has been grown and marketed in the U.S. for nearly 200 years, it remains an uncommon food. Despite its lack of popularity, it's actually a great-tasting vegetable with a delicate sweetness and flavor that hints of cabbage and turnip.

WHAT MAKES IT SO SPECIAL?

Rutabagas contain a wide spectrum of nutrients, including manganese, potassium, phosphorous, magnesium, and vitamin C. Rutabaga extract has been shown to inhibit proliferation and promote death of cancer cells.[1] Like other members of the cruciferous family, rutabagas are very high in fiber, providing more than 12 percent of your daily requirement in each one-cup serving. Rutabagas work well in soups or stews; they are also great on their own, baked or steamed as a side dish.

DID YOU KNOW...?

Rutabagas sold in supermarkets often are coated with a wax to increase their shelf life, so they should be peeled. For rutabagas from a farmer's market, you can peel or just scrub them before preparing.

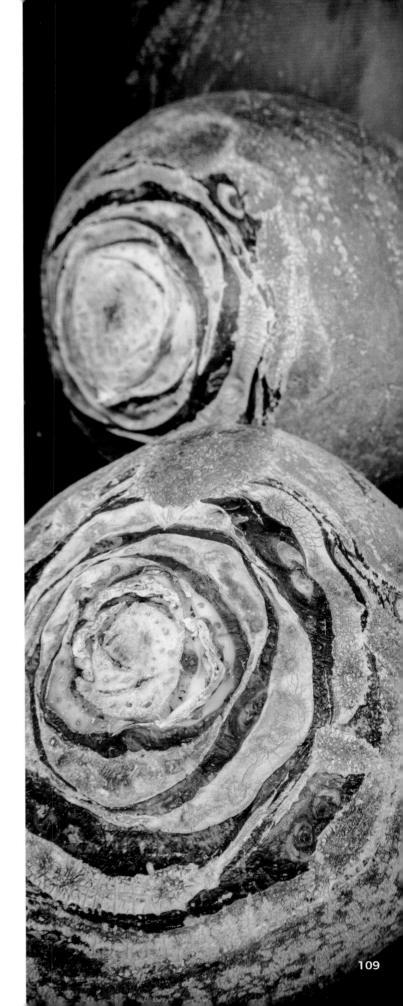

SCALLIONS

Scallions have been a popular herbal medicine in Asia for millennia. They were mentioned 2,000 years ago in *Shen Nong Ben Cao Jing*, the premodern classic Chinese book on agriculture and herbs.

WHAT MAKES THEM SO SPECIAL?

Scallions, also known as green onions, are young onions harvested when the bulbs are straight. They are often confused with spring onions, which have a small bulb at the base and are stronger in flavor. The entire scallion, including the stem, leaf and base, can be used raw in salads, added to stir-fries and sauces, or used as a garnish, to add a mild onion flavor to dishes. The onion family has powerful anticancer properties, but scallions are even more special, because they not only have thiosulfinates, but are also rich in minerals and vitamin K, and provide some carotenoids.[1]

LEEKS

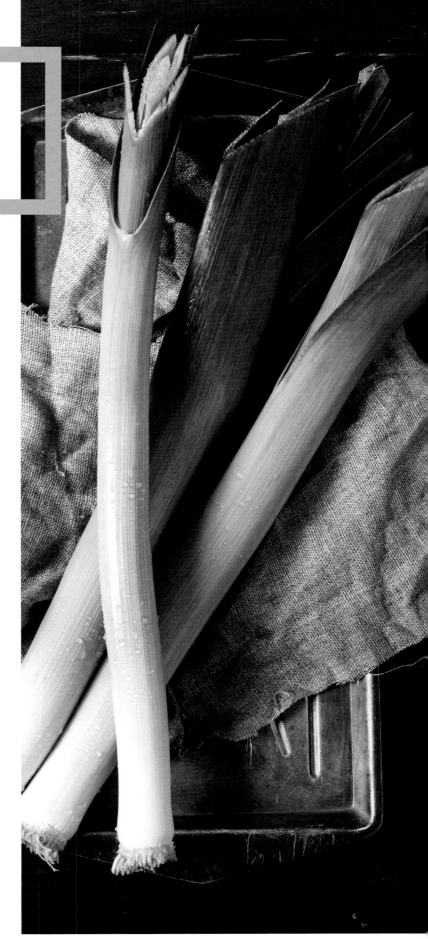

The leek is associated with the Welsh saint, David, who lived during the Middle Ages. Legend says that Welsh soldiers were instructed by St. David to wear leeks on their helmets in a battle against the Saxons, so they could easily identify other soldiers on their side. Leeks are the national symbol of Wales and are still worn there on St. David's Day (March 1).

WHAT MAKES THEM SO SPECIAL?

Leeks, like garlic, onions and scallions, belong to a genus of plants called Allium. These vegetables contain beneficial organosulfur compounds which have cancer-fighting actions.[1-3] They also have properties that inhibit the growth of harmful microorganisms.[4] Also present in leeks are impressive concentrations of flavonoid antioxidants which play a role in cardiovascular health, protecting our blood vessels from oxidative damage.[5, 6]

PREPARATION

Cleaning leeks can be a little tricky. Slice the leek lengthwise and peel apart each leaf to expose the dirt that somehow finds its way between its layers. Maximize the anti-cancer benefits of leeks by blending the entire leek when raw and then adding it to soups and stews for an excellent flavor boost.

SESAME SEEDS

Sesame, one of the oldest plants cultivated by humans, is believed to have originated in India or Africa, and is now grown all over the world. Sesame seed remains found in archeological excavations are thought to be from as far back as 3500-3050 B.C. Tahini, a paste of ground sesame seeds, is a staple in the cuisines of the eastern Mediterranean and Middle East.

WHAT MAKES THEM SO SPECIAL?

These little seeds are a goldmine of health benefits, and are an excellent source of essential minerals such as calcium, iron, manganese, magnesium, selenium and copper. Note that unhulled sesame seeds are richer in these minerals, especially calcium, compared to the more common hulled seeds. Sesame seeds are one of the few foods (along with flax and chia seeds) that contain lignans, phytochemicals with antioxidant and anti-estrogenic properties that are linked to a reduction in breast cancer risk.[1]

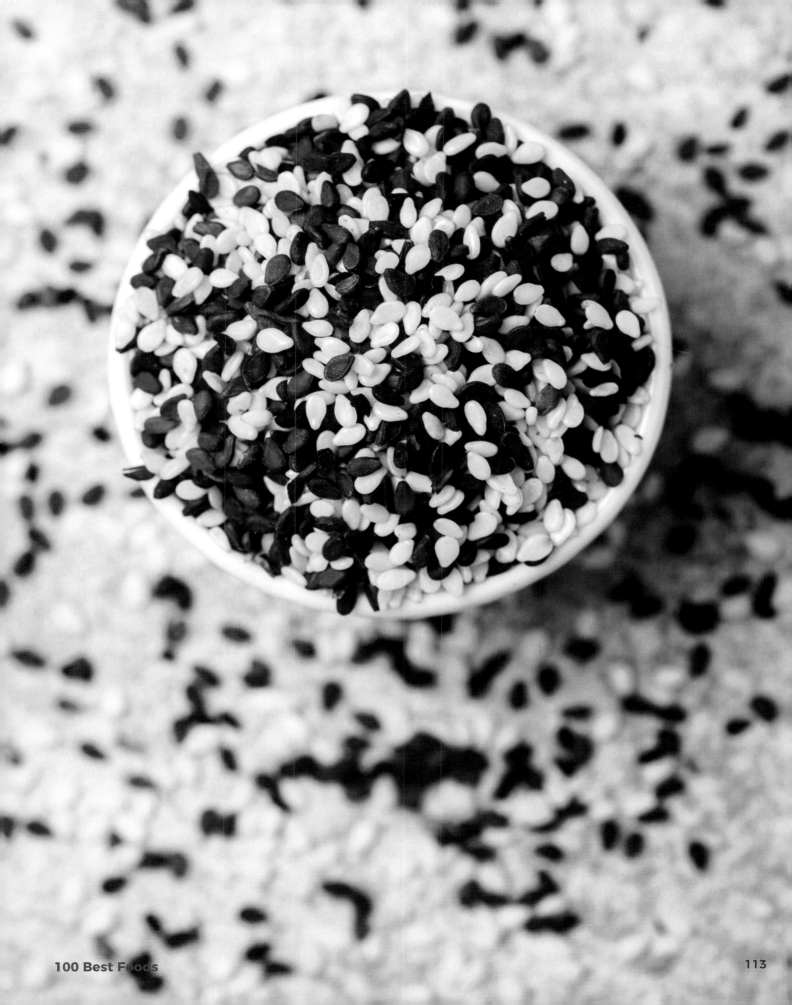

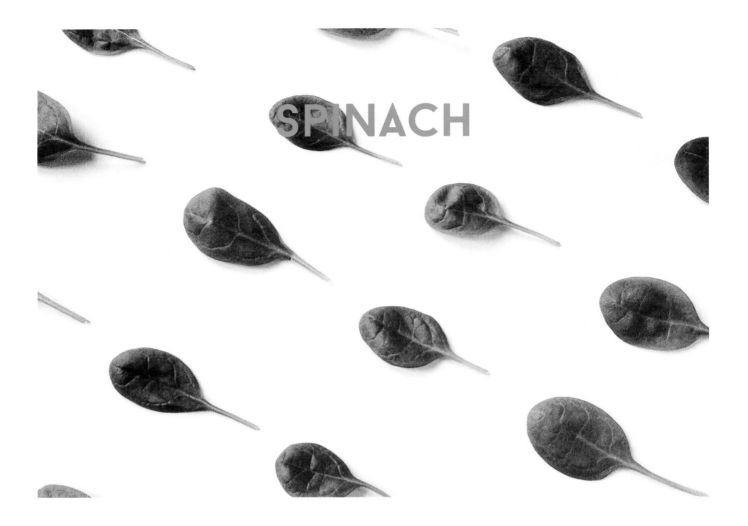

SPINACH

The word "Florentine" in food describes a dish served or prepared on a bed of spinach. This is attributed to Florence, Italy – the birthplace of Catherine de Medici, who married France's Prince Henry (later King Henry II) in 1533, and who is said to have introduced spinach into French cuisine.

WHAT MAKES IT SO SPECIAL?

Popeye sure knew what he was doing when he popped a can of spinach into his mouth to give him super strength to fight off the bad guys. Recent research has revealed that dietary nitrate, which is abundant in spinach and beets, may act as an athletic performance enhancer by enhancing blood flow. This property of spinach means it also may be beneficial for keeping blood pressure down and keeping the cardiovascular system healthy.[1-3] Spinach is high in vitamin K, which is important for bone health, and is also high in iron. This leafy green vegetable is one of the best sources of dietary magnesium, which is necessary for energy metabolism, maintaining muscle and nerve function, heart rhythm, a healthy immune system, and regulation of blood pressure.[4]

An important note about spinach: although it is an excellent food, don't make it the only leafy green you eat, because the calcium in spinach is not absorbable; kale, broccoli, bok choy, and collards have highly absorbable calcium.[5]

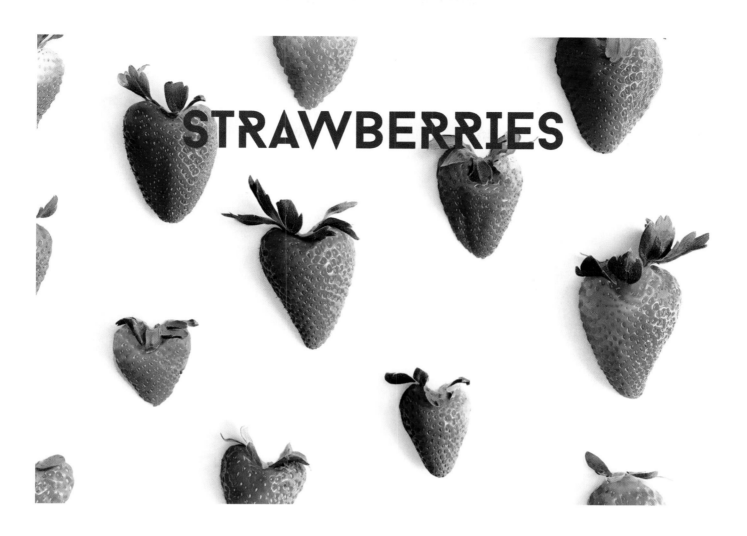

STRAWBERRIES

WHAT MAKES THEM SO SPECIAL?

The strawberry is considered one of the world's most popular berries; these juicy red fruits don't just look pretty and taste great, they have big health benefits backed up by many scientific studies. Higher strawberry intake is associated with reduced risk of death from cardiovascular disease.[1] Exploring the reasons why, several human trials have found that daily consumption of strawberries or strawberry powder has decreased total and LDL cholesterol, adhesion molecules, oxidized LDL, or measures of inflammation and oxidative stress.[2-10] Adding strawberries to a meal was also shown to reduce the insulin response in overweight adults in multiple studies, suggesting strawberries are a helpful food for people with diabetes or prediabetes.[6, 11] Even more impressive is the potential for strawberries to protect against cancer. In a Phase II clinical trial, patients with precancerous esophageal lesions ate freeze-dried strawberries each day for six months. The results were striking. Eighty percent of the patients in the high-dose strawberry group (60 grams/day) experienced a decrease in the histological grade of their lesion – this means that the progression toward cancer began to reverse.[12]

DID YOU KNOW...?

When buying strawberries, choose organic fruit whenever possible. Strawberries are routinely at or near the top of the Environmental Working Group's annual "Dirty Dozen" list, which points out the fruits and vegetables most likely to be contaminated by pesticides. If you are not buying organic, non-organic frozen strawberries are a better choice than non-organic fresh strawberries, as they are not sprayed with fungicides. Frozen berries of all types are considerably more affordable and highly recommended.

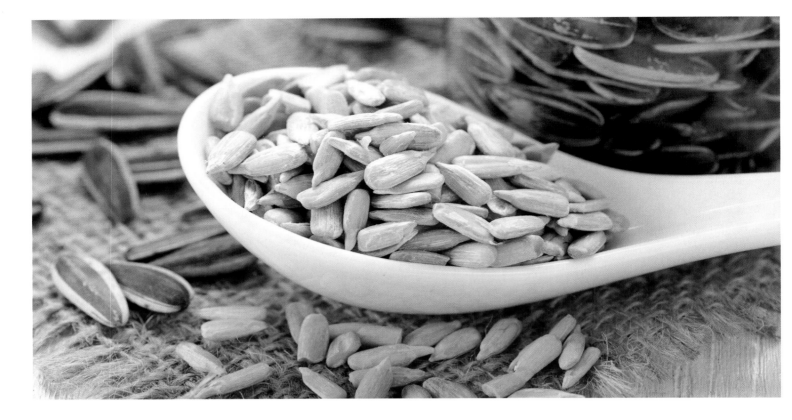

SUNFLOWER SEEDS

The sunflower has much more to it than its beauty: the bright yellow flower produces grayish-green or black seeds that have been used by Native Americans as both a food and a source of oil for more than 5,000 years. The Hopi Indians used the purplish-black seed hulls to create red and indigo dyes that were used in coloring grasses and other natural materials for basket weaving, clothing, and even face paint.

WHAT MAKES THEM SO SPECIAL?

Sunflowers are one of the few heliotropic plants – the young flowers turn their faces to follow the sun from east to west every day. Heliotropism is thought to aid in growth and photosynthesis. Sunflowers can grow up to 12 feet tall and 20 inches in diameter. These seeds are rich in protein and provide a natural spectrum of vitamin E compounds, supplying both tocopherols and tocotrienols – whereas, taking synthetic Vitamin E from supplements is dangerous.[1] Vitamin E's antioxidant properties reduce LDL cholesterol oxidation; it also reduces platelet aggregation, and its anti-inflammatory properties help prevent the development of atherosclerotic plaque.[2] Sunflower seeds provide extra cardiovascular protection because they are also rich in plant sterols, which help to reduce cholesterol levels.[3]

DID YOU KNOW...?

In the 1960s, baseball superstar Reggie Jackson chewed sunflower seeds during games instead of tobacco, sparking a healthful trend that continues to this day.

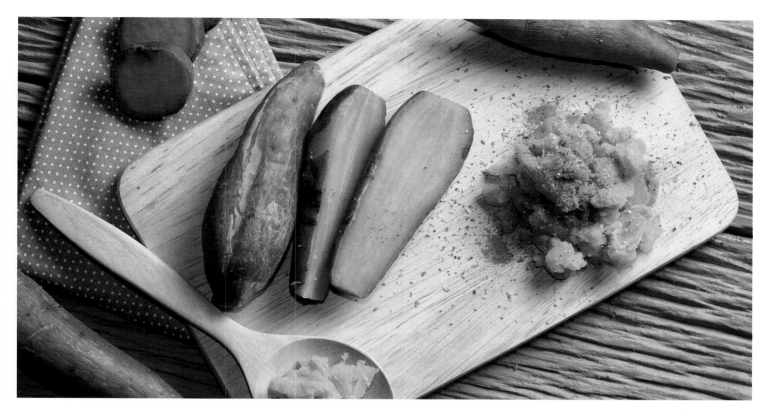

SWEET POTATOES

Sweet potatoes are native to Central and South America, and are one of the oldest vegetables known to man, dating back 2500-1850 B.C. They were brought to Spain by Christopher Columbus. The name "sweet potato" didn't show up until the 1740s, when it was used by American colonists to differentiate sweet potatoes from white potatoes. Today sweet potatoes are popular throughout the world.

WHAT MAKES THEM SO SPECIAL?

Sweet potatoes are rich in carotenes – especially beta-carotene, which is an important antioxidant and precursor to vitamin A.

Via beta-carotene, one medium sweet potato provides your body with four times the recommended daily allowance of vitamin A – an antioxidant vitamin that is crucial for the immune system, for vision, and is associated with a lower risk of macular degeneration.[1,2] Beta-carotene also helps to protect your skin from sun damage, by both deflecting and repairing oxidative cell damage caused by excessive UV exposure.[3,4] Sweet potatoes are rich in fiber and vitamin C, another potent antioxidant vitamin that plays an important role in preventing disease and enhancing longevity.

DID YOU KNOW...?

Sweet potatoes come in many varieties. Jewel is the orange-fleshed variety most familiar in the United States. Jewel sweet potatoes are often referred to as yams in the U.S., though they are actually sweet potatoes. Yams are generally drier and starchier.

SWISS CHARD

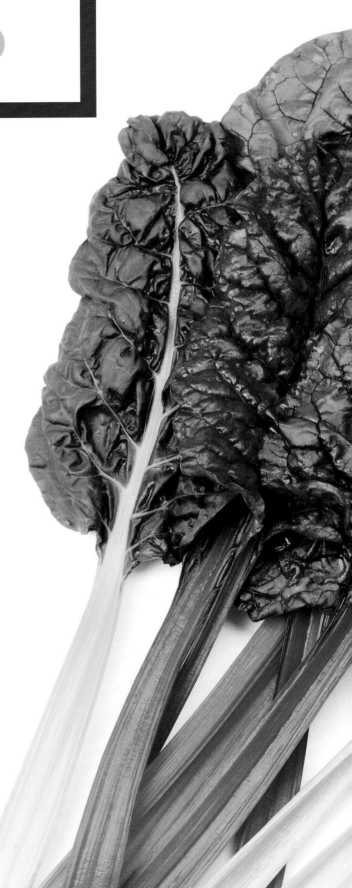

Swiss chard has been around for quite some time, revered by the ancient Greeks and the Romans for its medicinal properties. It is member of the beet family; however, unlike beets, the roots of Swiss chard are inedible.

WHAT MAKES IT SO SPECIAL?

Swiss chard is one of the richest food sources of lutein and zeaxanthin. These are carotenoids that protect the retina from sunlight and blue light damage, helping to preserve eye health and prevent Age-related Macular Degeneration (AMD).[1] Like other members of the beet family, Swiss chard is rich in phytochemicals known as betalains, which have powerful antioxidant and anti-inflammatory benefits. Also similar to beets, betalains give Swiss chard its characteristic deep red or yellow stems.[2] However, if you are prone to developing kidney stones, you may want to avoid consuming too much of this leafy green (especially raw). That's because it contains oxalate – a compound that binds calcium, limiting its absorption – and can be a factor in those prone to forming calcium oxalate kidney stones.

DID YOU KNOW...?

Despite its name, Swiss chard is not native to Switzerland; it actually originated in Sicily. As a result of its origin, Swiss chard continues to be a staple in Italian and Mediterranean cuisine.

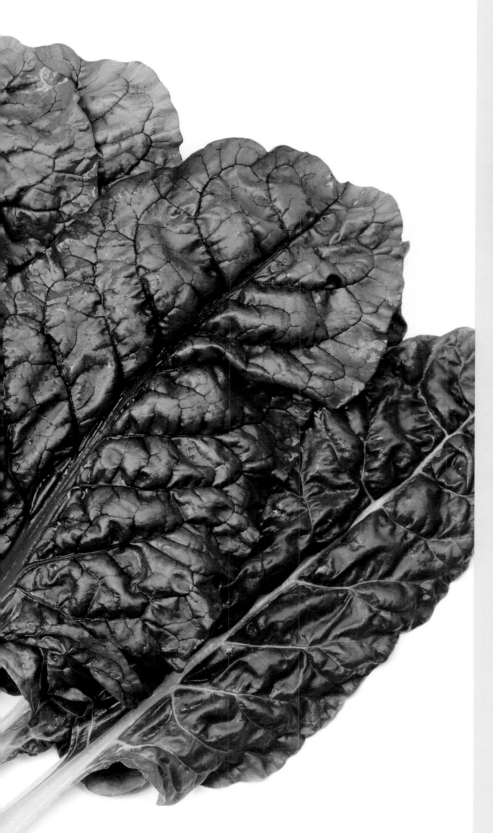

SWISS CHARD WITH ORANGE ZEST
SERVES: 4

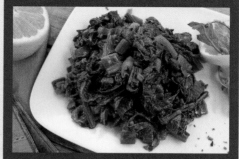

INGREDIENTS
2 bunches Swiss chard, stems and leaves separated and chopped
2 shallots, diced
2 cloves garlic, diced
1 organic orange, zested and juiced
1 pinch allspice
1 pinch chipotle chili flakes
1 tablespoon Dr. Fuhrman's Black Fig Vinegar or balsamic vinegar

INSTRUCTIONS
1. Sauté the shallots, garlic and swiss chard stems in a hot, dry stainless steel pan for 3-5 minutes, stirring constantly.

2. Add the orange zest and juice, allspice, and chipotle chili flakes.

3. Deglaze the pan with vinegar, then add the chard leaves and steam for 3 more minutes.

TOMATOES

Unbelievably, the tomato was unknown in the U.S. until long after it was commonly eaten in Europe. Not until after the Declaration of Independence was signed in 1776 do we find any record of the tomato being grown in this country. We sure did make up for it though: the U.S. is now one of the world's leading producers of both fresh and processed tomatoes.

WHAT MAKES THEM SO SPECIAL?

Tomatoes are the biggest source of dietary lycopene; a powerful antioxidant that, unlike some other nutrients in fruits and vegetables, is more easily absorbed by the body after cooking.[1,2] The antioxidant effects of lycopene help protect the skin from sun damage.[3] Lycopene also contains other protective mechanisms, such as anti-inflammatory and cholesterol-lowering actions.[4,5] Tomatoes are also rich in vitamins C and E, beta-carotene, and many flavonol antioxidants. Additionally, a relationship has been found between eating more tomatoes and a lower risk of certain cancers (especially prostate cancer) as well as heart attack, stroke, and hip fractures.[6-10]

DID YOU KNOW...?

Tomatoes should be kept at room temperature; refrigeration negatively affects their flavor and texture.

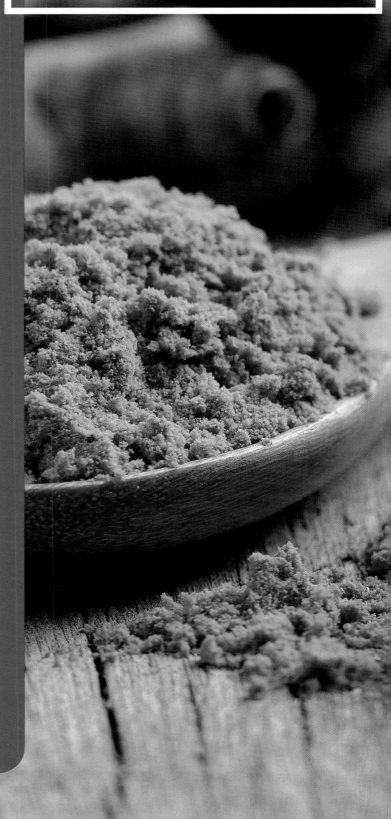

Archaeologists discovered pots near New Delhi with residue from turmeric, ginger, and garlic that date back as early as 2500 B.C. But it wasn't until about 500 B.C. that turmeric emerged as an important part of Ayurvedic medicine, an ancient Indian system of natural healing. Although this yellow spice has had culinary and medicinal uses for over 4,500 years, only in recent years has it been widely recognized for its health benefits.

TURMERIC

WHAT MAKES IT SO SPECIAL?

The main active ingredient in turmeric is curcumin (a collective name for a group of phytochemicals called curcuminoids), which is known for its potent anti-inflammatory effects.[1] In human studies, curcumin supplementation has resulted in measurable reductions in inflammatory markers, such as C-reactive protein.[2] Curcumin and other turmeric phytochemicals, such as tumerones, have been shown in studies to have anti-cancer effects including scavenging free radicals, blocking inflammatory signals, and inhibiting the growth and proliferation of cancerous cells.[3-5] Curcumin's anti-inflammatory properties have been tested for their ability to reduce inflammation associated with osteoarthritis.[6, 7] This super spice also helps keep your skin healthy; there is evidence that curcumin inhibits the growth of pimple-causing bacteria on the skin.[8] As a seasoning, turmeric can add delicious complexity to mashed dishes like potatoes or cauliflower, or sauté it with onions, broccoli, carrots, or bell peppers. It can also be used in vegetable dips and sauces.

DID YOU KNOW...?

Be sure to buy the full, organic turmeric spice rather than getting it as part of a spice blend, like in a curry powder. You'll get more of the curcumin and other beneficial phytochemicals if you use turmeric itself.

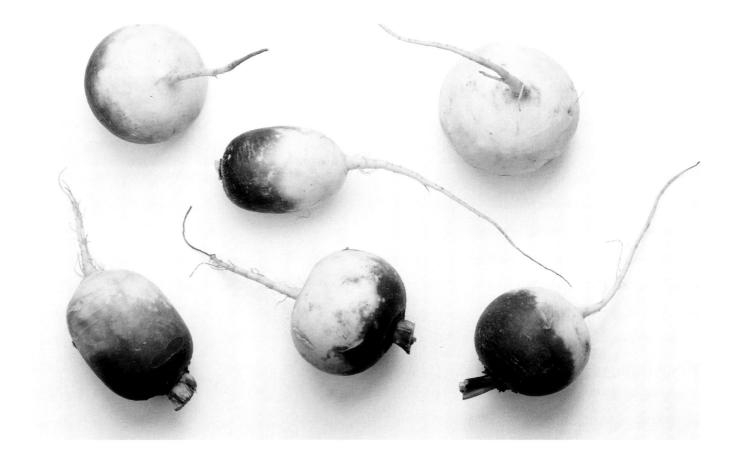

TURNIPS

Turnips have gotten a bad rap in the past; it is said that Romans used to throw turnips at unpopular people. It was believed that turnips were only for those who were either poor or starving, since they have consistently been a popular food for livestock. Times have changed however, and these days many people enjoy baked, steamed and even raw turnips.

WHAT MAKES THEM SO SPECIAL?

Turnips are members of the cruciferous vegetable family, known for their cancer-fighting compounds.[1] A one-cup serving of turnips supplies about one-third of the daily recommended vitamin C, and 3 grams of fiber. The leafy green tops are packed with even more nutrients than the white roots. When buying turnips, choose those that are younger and smaller (less than 3 inches wide) – smaller turnips can be sliced and added raw to salads, and are more tender with a very mild taste. Larger turnips may have tougher flesh and taste somewhat bitter. Young turnip greens can be eaten raw in salad, while older ones should be briefly steamed or water sautéed.

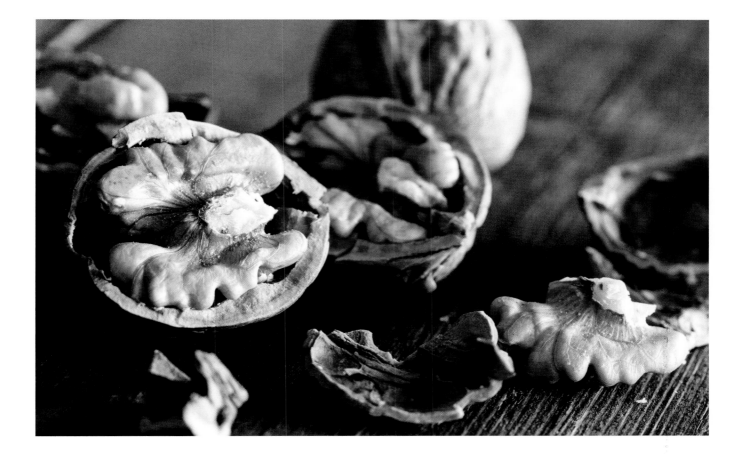

WALNUTS

Walnuts have been around for a long, long time – they were grown in King Solomon's garden circa 950 B.C. Today, California is responsible for 99 percent of the commercial United States supply, and about 75 percent of the entire world's supply. As the healthiest nut, I bestow upon them the title, the King of Nuts.

WHAT MAKES THEM SO SPECIAL?

Walnuts are an excellent source of polyphenols and the omega-3 fat alpha-linolenic acid (ALA), and are associated with potential benefits to both brain and heart health. Walnuts are linked to better brain function and improved memory.[1] Eating walnuts may counter age-related decline and reduce one's risk of neurodegenerative diseases, such as Alzheimer's disease.[2, 3] Alpha-linolenic acid, a plant-derived omega-3 fatty acid, is the precursor to DHA and EPA, important fatty acids in the brain.[4] Walnuts have been shown to reduce LDL cholesterol oxidation and have anti-inflammatory effects.[5, 6] Also, like all nuts, walnuts are strongly associated with living longer, staving off heart disease, and helping with weight loss and weight maintenance.[7-10]

DID YOU KNOW...?

Walnuts aid in your body's absorption of beneficial carotenoids when eaten along with other foods.

WATERCRESS PESTO PITAS

SERVES: 4

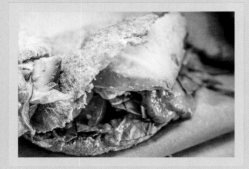

INGREDIENTS FOR THE PESTO

1 bulb garlic
2 cups watercress, stems removed
5 basil leaves
1/2 cup walnuts
4 tablespoons unsweetened soy,
hemp or almond milk

INGREDIENTS FOR THE SANDWICH

4 100% whole grain pitas
1 tomato, sliced
1/2 cup thinly sliced red onion
2 cups arugula
2 cups spinach
1 avocado, pit removed, sliced

INSTRUCTIONS

1. Slice bottom edge including root off garlic bulb. Lightly roast bulb for 15 minutes at 300 degrees F.

2. Cut open cloves and squeeze out soft, cooked garlic. Combine the roasted garlic with the other pesto ingredients in a high-powered blender until smooth.

3. Spread pesto on whole grain pitas. Stuff pita with the remaining sandwich ingredients.

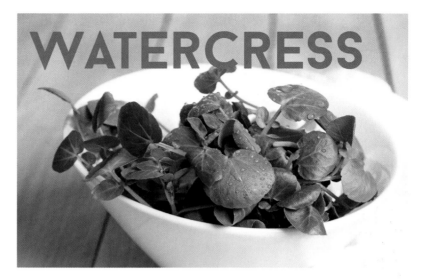

WATERCRESS

This ancient, peppery-flavored green is believed to have been a staple in the diet of Roman soldiers. Hippocrates, the father of medicine, used watercress to treat his patients.

WHAT MAKES IT SO SPECIAL?

As one of the healthiest foods in the world, everyone could get lifespan benefits by adding watercress to their diet. Watercress is a cruciferous leafy green that contains a powerhouse of nutrients. It is rich in vitamins C and K, as well as antioxidant phytochemicals lutein and zeaxanthin. Lutein and zeaxanthin are carotenoids that protect the eyes against damage from sunlight.[1] Rutin, a flavonoid contained in watercress leaves, is a bone-building nutrient. Rutin-rich watercress extract improved the growth and proliferation of osteoblasts (bone-building cells) in vitro, as well as collagen production and mineralization, two other important properties of these cells.[2] Another important phytochemical in watercress is a glucosinolate called gluconasturtiin, which is a precursor to the ITC phenethyl isothiocyanate (PEITC). ITCs are cancer-fighting phytochemicals derived from cruciferous vegetables. Research has revealed that the PEITC in watercress has the ability to suppress breast cancer cell development by "turning off" an angiogenic signal from cancerous cells, thereby preventing the tumor from getting the blood supply it needs to grow. In one study, four breast cancer survivors ingested 80 grams of watercress (about 2 cups). A few hours later, blood PEITC levels were elevated, and the angiogenic signal of interest was reduced.[3, 4] Another study on healthy men showed that supplementing the diet with watercress helped to limit DNA damage and oxidative stress following strenuous exercise.[5]

There's evidence that this refreshing melon was cultivated in Egypt and Libya at least 4,000 years ago. Watermelon seeds were found in the tomb of Pharaoh Tutankhamun – otherwise known as "King Tut."

WHAT MAKES IT SO SPECIAL?

One of watermelon's many health benefits is that it is rich in the amino acid citrulline, which helps to keep blood pressure down. Studies on people with prehypertension or hypertension showed that watermelon extract supplements produced improvements in blood pressure compared to the placebo groups.[1, 2] Like tomatoes, watermelon is a rich source of lycopene, a very potent carotenoid antioxidant.[3] Lycopene has been shown to protect against prostate cancer, as well as protect the skin from the sun's rays. It also aids the cardiovascular system – higher lycopene levels in the blood are linked to a lower risk of heart attack and stroke.[4-7] Look for a melon that is dark green, heavy for its size, and uniform in shape. Next, look for a creamy yellow spot, known as the field spot. This is where the melon sat on the ground and ripened in the sun. The deeper the color, the longer the melon has been ripening, and the sweeter it has likely become. If the field spot is white or even non-existent, the watermelon was probably picked too early, and will never fully ripen.

WATERMELON

DID YOU KNOW...?

The citrulline in watermelon may also reduce muscle soreness after exercise. One study found that athletes who were given 16 ounces of watermelon juice after a bout of intense exercise had lower levels of muscle soreness 24 hours later, compared to athletes given a placebo drink.[8]

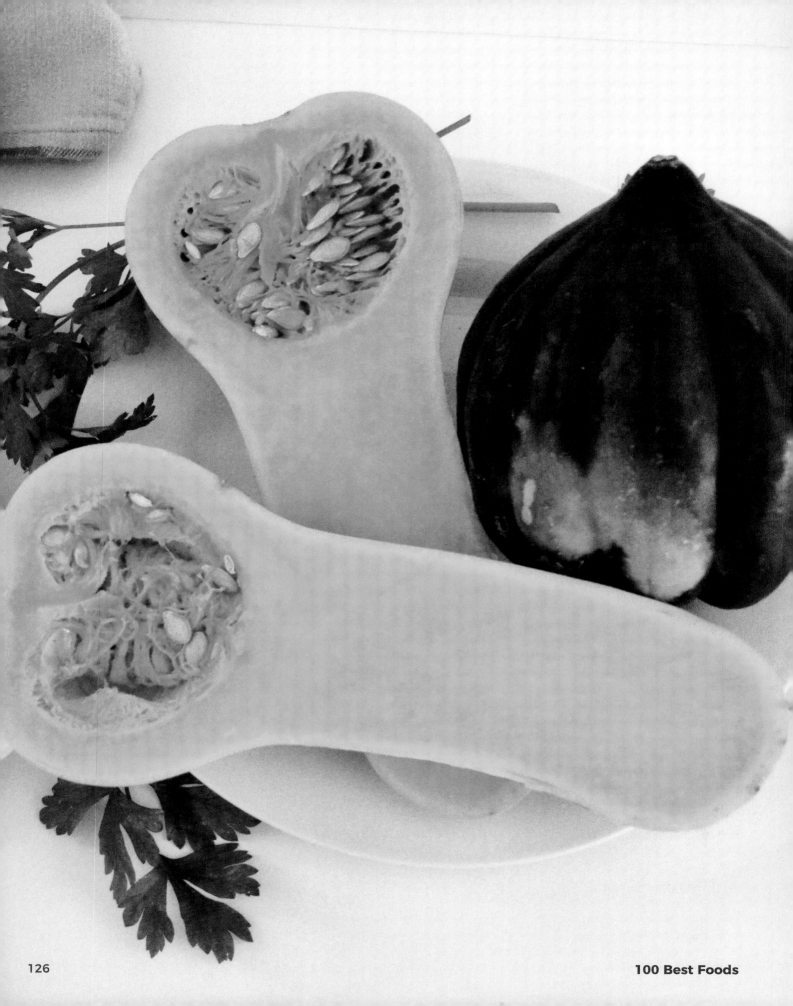

WINTER SQUASH

Make sure you have a lot of room in your garden if you plant winter squash – the sprawling vines of some varieties can grow anywhere from 10 to 20 feet long. Butternut, buttercup, acorn, pumpkin, delicata, hubbard, spaghetti squash and more are available from late fall through the winter.

WHAT MAKES IT SO SPECIAL?

Squashes are special because they can be picked in late summer and retain their flavor and nutrients while in storage for months. Thanks to this property, they have been supplying us with fresh vegetables throughout the winter for thousands of years. The yellow and orange colors of winter squash are an indicator of its particularly rich supply of alpha-carotene, beta-carotene and beta-cryptoxanthin. These carotenoids provide us with vitamin A and offer protection against aging and chronic diseases by preventing oxidative damage. Carotenoids counteract UV-induced oxidative stress in the skin, and have been shown to prevent or repair DNA damage to the skin caused by the sun.[1,2] High blood levels of circulating carotenoids have been linked to longer life.[3]

DID YOU KNOW...?

The wording on that can of "100 percent pumpkin puree" in your pantry might be misleading. According to the USDA, other "clean, sound, properly matured, golden-fleshed, firm-shelled, sweet varieties of either pumpkins and squashes" are acceptable substitutes, and can be labeled as 100 percent pumpkin.

ACORN SQUASH SUPREME
SERVES: 2

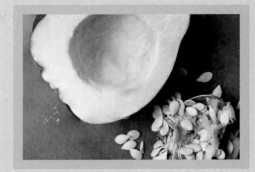

INGREDIENTS
1 large acorn or butternut squash
1/4 cup dried unsulfured apricots, soaked in just enough water to almost cover until soft, then diced
1 1/2 cups pineapple, chopped
2 tablespoons raisins
2 tablespoons chopped walnuts
cinnamon

INSTRUCTIONS
1. Preheat oven to 350 degrees F .

2. Cut squash in half, remove seeds, and bake face down in ½ inch of water for 45 minutes.

2. Meanwhile, combine the apricots and soaking liquid, pineapple, raisins, and walnuts.

3. After the squash has cooked, scoop the fruit/nut mixture into the squash's center. Place in pan and cover loosely with aluminum foil.

4. Bake for an additional 30 minutes. Sprinkle with cinnamon, then put it back in the oven for 5 more minutes.

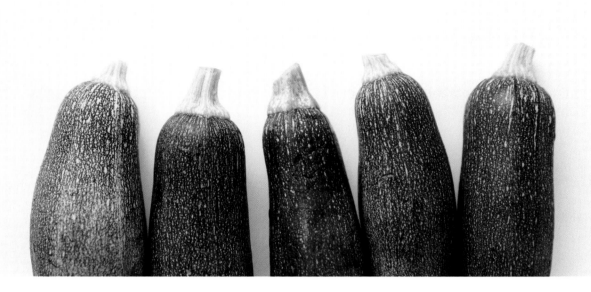

ZUCCHINI

Zucchini is the most familiar cultivar of summer squash, a long, cylindrical green vegetable (though botanically, it can be considered a fruit). The earliest records of squash date from the early 16th century in France, Italy, and the Americas. Zucchini itself started showing up in Italian cookbooks during the 19th century. The name zucchini comes from the Italian word "zucca," meaning squash, plus "-ini," the plural form of the suffix meaning little.[1]

WHAT MAKES IT SO SPECIAL?

A perfect weight loss food, zucchini is low in calories but high in fiber, beta-carotene, lutein and zeaxanthin, potassium, manganese, and vitamin C. Zucchini gives you a full feeling after eating due to its high water and fiber content. A diet high in potassium and low in sodium can help keep blood pressure down; beta carotene is a powerful antioxidant; and lutein and zeaxanthin help protect the retina from light damage.[2, 3] When buying zucchini, look for ones that are sleek, smooth and firm, with bright-colored skin. Bigger is not better in this case – large zucchini can be tough and seedy; small to medium ones (approximately 6-8 inches) usually have a better flavor. When preparing, do not remove the skin, because it contains much of the favorable anti-cancer compounds.

DID YOU KNOW...?

One cup of cooked zucchini has just as much potassium as a medium-size banana.

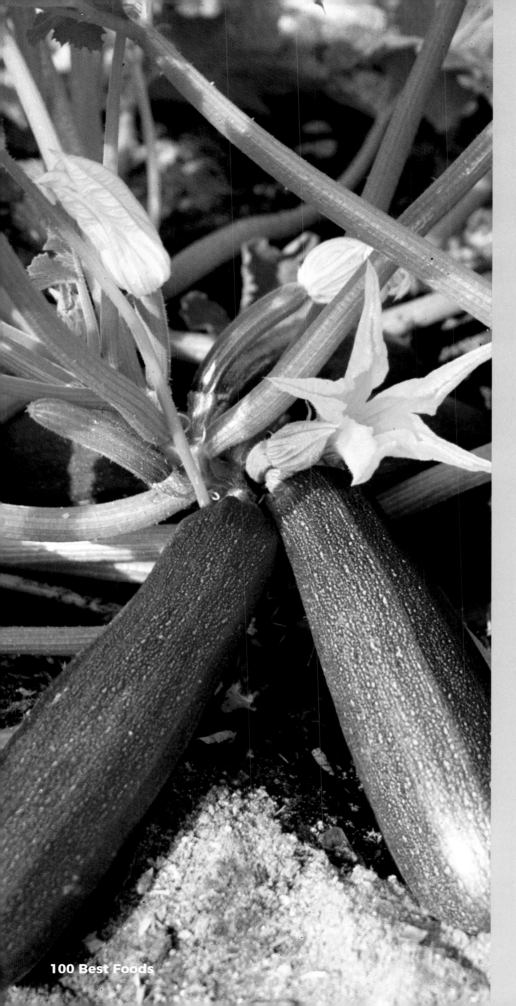

ZUCCHINI SPAGHETTI
SERVES: 4

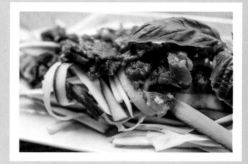

INGREDIENTS

3 medium zucchini, cut to resemble spaghetti (see note)
1/2 large sweet onion, chopped
5 garlic cloves, chopped
4 ounces mushrooms, sliced
4 medium tomatoes, chopped
4 basil leaves, chopped

INSTRUCTIONS

1. After cutting the zucchini, let it drain in a colander.

2. While zucchini is draining, heat 2 tablespoons water in a sauté pan and sauté onion until tender, about 5 minutes. Add garlic and cook for 30 seconds or until fragrant. Add the mushrooms and cook until softened and tender. Add the tomatoes and basil and cook for another 5 minutes.

3. Serve zucchini topped with the tomato sauce.

Note: A vegetable spiralizer works well for cutting the zucchini.

FOOD FOR THOUGHT

Learn how the Nutritarian Diet incorporates the best foods on the planet

Now that you know the 100 best foods for health and longevity, the next step is to learn how to incorporate them into an eating plan that is logical, sustainable, healthful, and – most of all – delicious. That is the basis of my Nutritarian Diet – an eating style consisting of high-nutrient, whole plant foods that supply a copious amount of micronutrients. This unleashes the body's tremendous ability to heal, achieve optimal weight and slow the aging process. Following this healthful diet will allow you to break away from eating foods loaded with addictive substances like sugar, salt, oil and white flour.

FEED YOUR MIND

What follows is a brief overview of the principles of the Nutritarian diet, and a plan for helping you to get started. But to achieve long-term success in your health and weight loss journey, you will need to learn the critical facts about nutritional excellence. I strongly suggest that you read one or more of my books, and take advantage of the information available on my website, www.DrFuhrman.com; you can even become an expert by studying at our Nutritarian Education Institute.

Remember: knowledge is stronger than willpower. When you are armed with the right information, you have the best opportunity to remove cravings, end yo-yo dieting and avoid emotional overeating. Educating yourself, and then enlisting the right support will aid in your enjoyment and success.

THE SCIENCE

The key to optimizing your health and achieving an ideal body weight is to eat food with a relatively high proportion of micronutrients to calories. Micronutrients (which do not contain calories) consist of vitamins, minerals and phytochemicals. Macronutrients (which contain calories) consist of fat, carbohydrate and protein. Most Americans are deficient in micronutrients, and consume too many macronutrients.

Natural, colorful plant foods have the greatest amount (and widest assortment) of micronutrients, including those anti-cancer phytonutrients. Eating more high-nutrient plant food crowds out both unhealthy foods and those with a higher caloric density.

DR. FUHRMAN
Products

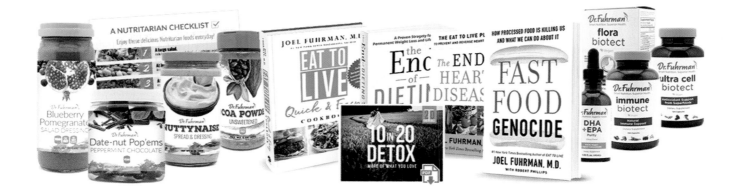

At DrFuhrman.com, we offer a wide range of high-quality supplements, food products, books and more that can help to support your health and wellness goals.

Dr. Fuhrman's line of nutrition bars, salad dressings, soups, sauces and other products are made with whole foods, and do not contain salt, oil or artificial sweeteners. Be sure to check out our Nutrition Facts information, to see how low in sugar these products are – making them a great choice for those looking to lose weight and achieve incredible health.

The premium supplements in Dr. Fuhrman's line are carefully designed to supply the important vitamins and nutrients your body needs, without ingredients like folic acid or vitamin A, which can be dangerous in supplemental form.

Dr. Fuhrman's books, which include the New York Times bestsellers *Eat to Live*, *The End of Dieting*, *The End of Heart Disease*, and *Super Immunity* and his groundbreaking work, *Fast Food Genocide*, will help you gain expert-level knowledge in the science of nutrition.

100 Best Foods

BECOME A MEMBER OF DRFUHRMAN.COM

Your recipe for success!

LEARN HOW FOOD AFFECTS YOUR HEALTH

Knowing the Top 100 Foods is helpful, but it is only the beginning. To achieve optimal health, you need to know how to make high-nutrient, whole plant foods the foundation of your daily diet.

Joel Fuhrman, M.D. created his website to educate, support and inspire. DrFuhrman.com is your one-stop source for information on how to eat better, prevent and reverse disease, and slow the aging process.

As a member, you'll gain access to . . .

- Articles and videos focusing on nutritional science and a healthy lifestyle
- Over 1,600 delicious Nutritarian Recipes, with shopping lists
- A Health Tracker to track your progress and store your important health information
- Online member communities
- Ask the Doctor and Ask the Food Addiction Specialist discussions
- Targeted meal plans
- Exclusive Facebook Live presentations
- Members-only magazine
- Generous product discounts

DrFuhrman.com . . .
The roadmap to a healthier version of you!

Visit www.DrFuhrman.com/membership
or call Customer Service at 1 (800) 474-WELL (9355)

YOUR SIX-WEEK PATH TO NUTRITIONAL EXCELLENCE

WEEK 2

Week 2
EAT A LARGE RAW SALAD AS A MAIN DISH EVERY DAY FOR LUNCH OR DINNER.

Now is the time to begin flooding your body with raw vegetables, the most powerful anti-cancer, longevity-promoting foods in the world. Use lettuce and tomatoes, but don't forget the raw cruciferous veggies shredded on top, plus onions, scallions and, of course, a healthy dressing made with nuts and seeds. I have scores of fantastic dressing recipes on DrFuhrman.com and in my books. For those too busy to make their own, we offer some no-salt dressings made from nuts, seeds and other whole foods packaged in glass bottles to make your life easy. A big daily salad is the secret fountain of youth.

WEEK 1

Week 3
GOT BEAN SOUP?

Make a giant pot of vegetable-bean soup, stew or chili every weekend, and portion it out into many single-serving containers to use all week long. Make sure this soup includes beans, lentils or split peas, mushrooms and onion, and has a vegetable broth base made with real vegetable juices. Season it with herbs and spices, but no salt. Try some of my fantastic soup recipes and over time, find your top four that you will make most of the time. Now you can have a salad and soup for lunch, with one fresh fruit for dessert. You are two-thirds on your way to being a full-fledged Nutritarian. See how easy this was?

WEEK 3

Week 1
GET RID OF JUNK FOOD, HIGH-GLYCEMIC CARBOHYDRATES AND FRIED FOODS

To be successful, you must commit to this plan 100 percent — that means no fried foods, no processed foods, no white flour, no sugar or other sweeteners. Do not use honey or maple syrup; foods can be sweetened only with fruit and non-sulfured dried fruits, such as dates. You may experience headaches for a few days, or feel unwell. This is a sign that the toxins are leaving your system. Start reading my books this first week. Pick two books to read, depending on your interest, and go through them with a highlighter, marking those sections that are important to your life. I recommend starting with **The End of Dieting** or **Eat For Health.**

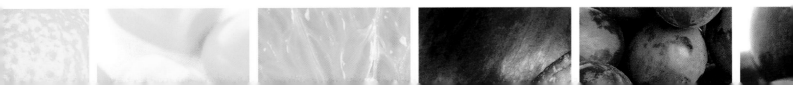

WEEK 4

Week 4
NUTRITARIAN-IZE YOUR BREAKFAST

Add one tablespoon of ground chia or flax seeds with one tablespoon of hemp seeds to an intact grain cooked in water, such as steel-cut oats, quinoa, buckwheat, kasha or millet. Don't forget to add the berries – frozen is fine. Unsweetened soy, almond or hemp milk can be used, too. Now you have G-BOMBS in your diet. (You are almost a full-fledged Nutritarian now.)
Another Nutritarian breakfast option is a green smoothie, made with berries and seeds.

DR. FUHRMAN'S HEALTH EQUATION:

H=N/C

Your long-term Health is predicted by your Nutrient intake, per Calorie eaten

WEEK 6

Week 6
REDUCE OR ELIMINATE ANIMAL PRODUCTS, AND ELIMINATE OIL AND SALT

Now is the time to practice animal protein restriction – this is an anti-aging technique that also defends against cancer. Your breakfast and lunch are already set; they are Nutritarian and vegan. But don't use more than 2 ounces of animal products with any dinner. And if you had some animal-based food one evening, make the next day completely vegan, so you are only consuming one or two ounces of animal products, every other day.

Now is also the time to get all the oil out of your diet, except for very small amounts. Your only concentrated fat source will now come from nuts and seeds. And make sure you have reduced the sodium in your diet to a maximum of 1000 mg a day. The natural sodium in whole natural foods will be about 400 to 600 mg a day, so that means not more than 400 mg of sodium a day from any added source, such a tomato sauce or whole grain bread.

WEEK 5

Week 5
EAT YOUR GREENS (AND OTHER COOKED VEGETABLES!)

This week you will include a large serving of cooked greens and other vegetables every dinner as a main dish. In addition to prepping your bountiful salad every day, you will also need to spend some time at the stove, so there are a few cooking techniques you'll need to master. Water sautéing is great for creating stir-fries: place a quarter cup of water in a very hot pan, add chopped vegetables, and stir for about 5 minutes, until the vegetables start to soften. Then add a few table-spoons of a delicious sauce, such as spicy red sauce or a creamy and savory nut sauce. My favorite is my Thai Curry Sauce, which makes any vegetable mixture taste like gourmet fare.

Quick and easy tip: use frozen veggies instead of fresh to decrease prep time.

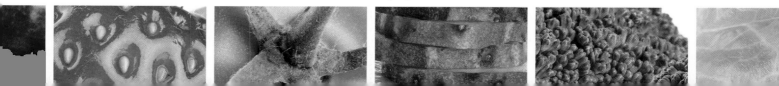

Almonds

1. Kris-Etherton PM, Hu FB, Ros E, Sabate J. The role of tree nuts and peanuts in the prevention of coronary heart disease: multiple potential mechanisms. J Nutr 2008, 138:1746S-1751S.

2. Choudhury K, Clark J, Griffiths HR. An almond-enriched diet increases plasma alpha-tocopherol and improves vascular function but does not affect oxidative stress markers or lipid levels. Free Radic Res 2014, 48:599-606.

3. Jenkins DJ, Kendall CW, Marchie A, et al. Almonds reduce biomarkers of lipid peroxidation in older hyperlipidemic subjects. J Nutr 2008, 138:908-913.

4. Jenkins DJ, Kendall CW, Josse AR, et al. Almonds decrease postprandial glycemia, insulinemia, and oxidative damage in healthy individuals. J Nutr 2006, 136:2987-2992.

5. Jenkins DJ, Kendall CW, Marchie A, et al. Dose response of almonds on coronary heart disease risk factors: blood lipids, oxidized low-density lipoproteins, lipoprotein(a), homocysteine, and pulmonary nitric oxide: a randomized, controlled, crossover trial. Circulation 2002, 106:1327-1332.

6. Musa-Veloso K, Paulionis L, Poon T, Lee HY. The effects of almond consumption on fasting blood lipid levels: a systematic review and meta-analysis of randomised controlled trials. J Nutr Sci 2016, 5:e34.

7. Li SC, Liu YH, Liu JF, et al. Almond consumption improved glycemic control and lipid profiles in patients with type 2 diabetes mellitus. Metabolism 2011, 60:474-479.

8. Josse AR, Kendall CW, Augustin LS, et al. Almonds and postprandial glycemia—a dose-response study. Metabolism 2007, 56:400-404.

9. Jenkins DJ, Kendall CW, Marchie A, et al. Effect of almonds on insulin secretion and insulin resistance in nondiabetic hyperlipidemic subjects: a randomized controlled crossover trial. Metabolism 2008, 57:882-887.

10. Gulati S, Misra A, Pandey RM. Effect of Almond Supplementation on Glycemia and Cardiovascular Risk Factors in Asian Indians in North India with Type 2 Diabetes Mellitus: A 24-Week Study. Metab Syndr Relat Disord 2017, 15:98-105.

Apples

1. Koutsos A, Tuohy KM, Lovegrove JA. Apples and cardiovascular health—is the gut microbiota a core consideration? Nutrients 2015, 7:3959-3998.

2. Brown L, Rosner B, Willett WW, Sacks FM. Cholesterol-lowering effects of dietary fiber: a meta-analysis. Am J Clin Nutr 1999, 69:30-42.

3. Song Y, Manson JE, Buring JE, et al. Associations of dietary flavonoids with risk of type 2 diabetes, and markers of insulin resistance and systemic inflammation in women: a prospective study and cross-sectional analysis. J Am Coll Nutr 2005, 24:376-384.

4. Fabiani R, Minelli L, Rosignoli P. Apple intake and cancer risk: a systematic review and meta-analysis of observational studies. Public Health Nutr 2016, 19:2603-2617.

Apricots

1. Higdon J, Drake VJ: Fiber. In An Evidence-based Approach to Phytochemicals and Other Dietary Factors New York: Thieme; 2013: 133-148

2. Sochor J, Zitka O, Skutkova H, et al. Content of phenolic compounds and antioxidant capacity in fruits of apricot genotypes. Molecules 2010, 15:6285-6305.

Artichokes

1. Costabile A, Kolida S, Klinder A, et al. A double-blind, placebo-controlled, cross-over study to establish the bifidogenic effect of a very-long-chain inulin extracted from globe artichoke (Cynara scolymus) in healthy human subjects. Br J Nutr 2010, 104:1007-1017.

2. Sonnenburg ED, Sonnenburg JL. Starving our microbial self: the deleterious consequences of a diet deficient in microbiota-accessible carbohydrates. Cell Metab 2014, 20:779-786.

Arugula

1. Azarenko O, Jordan MA, Wilson L. Erucin, the major isothiocyanate in arugula (Eruca sativa), inhibits proliferation of MCF7 tumor cells by suppressing microtubule dynamics. PLoS One 2014, 9:e100599.

2. Cho HJ, Lee KW, Park JH. Erucin exerts anti-inflammatory properties in murine macrophages and mouse skin: possible mediation through the inhibition of NFkappaB signaling. Int J Mol Sci 2013, 14:20564-20577.

3. Alqasoumi S, Al-Sohaibani M, Al-Howiriny T, et al. Rocket "Eruca sativa": a salad herb with potential gastric anti-ulcer activity. World J Gastroenterol 2009, 15:1958-1965. Asparagus

Asparagus

1. Stolzenberg-Solomon RZ, Chang SC, Leitzmann MF, et al. Folate intake, alcohol use, and postmenopausal breast cancer risk in the Prostate, Lung, Colorectal, and Ovarian Cancer Screening Trial. Am J Clin Nutr 2006, 83:895-904.

2. Sanjoaquin MA, Allen N, Couto E, et al. Folate intake and colorectal cancer risk: a meta-analytical approach. Int J Cancer 2005, 113:825-828.

3.Smith AD, Kim YI, Refsum H. Is folic acid good for everyone? Am J Clin Nutr 2008, 87:517-533.

4. Mason JB, Dickstein A, Jacques PF, et al. A temporal association between folic acid fortification and an increase in colorectal cancer rates may be illuminating important biological principles: a hypothesis. Cancer Epidemiol Biomarkers Prev 2007, 16:1325-1329.

5. Drinkwater JM, Tsao R, Liu R, et al. Effects of cooking on rutin and glutathione concentrations and antioxidant activity of green asparagus (Asparagus officinalis) spears. Journal of Func-

tional Foods 2015, 12:342-353.

6.USDA Database for the Flavonoid Content of Selected Foods, Release 3 (2011) [http://www.ars.usda.gov/Services/docs.htm?docid=6231]

7.Marunaka Y, Marunaka R, Sun H, et al. Actions of Quercetin, a Polyphenol, on Blood Pressure. Molecules 2017, 22.

Avocado

1. Fulgoni VL, 3rd, Dreher M, Davenport AJ. Avocado consumption is associated with better diet quality and nutrient intake, and lower metabolic syndrome risk in US adults: results from the National Health and Nutrition Examination Survey (NHANES) 2001-2008. Nutr J 2013, 12:1.

2. Peou S, Milliard-Hasting B, Shah SA. Impact of avocado-enriched diets on plasma lipoproteins: A meta-analysis. J Clin Lipidol 2016, 10:161-171.

3. Wien M, Haddad E, Oda K, Sabate J. A randomized 3x3 crossover study to evaluate the effect of Hass avocado intake on post-ingestive satiety, glucose and insulin levels, and subsequent energy intake in overweight adults. Nutr J 2013, 12:155.

4. Dreher ML, Davenport AJ. Hass avocado composition and potential health effects. Crit Rev Food Sci Nutr 2013, 53:738-750.

Bananas

1. Sonnenburg ED, Sonnenburg JL. Starving our microbial self: the deleterious consequences of a diet deficient in microbiota-accessible carbohydrates. Cell Metab 2014, 20:779-786.

2. Hamer HM, Jonkers D, Venema K, et al. Review article: the role of butyrate on colonic function. Aliment Pharmacol Ther 2008, 27:104-119.

Basil

1. Kim IS, Yang MR, Lee OH, Kang SN. Antioxidant activities of hot water extracts from various spices. Int J Mol Sci 2011, 12:4120-4131.

2. Tenore GC, Campiglia P, Ciampaglia R, et al. Antioxidant and antimicrobial properties of traditional green and purple "Napoletano" basil cultivars (Ocimum basilicum L.) from Campania region (Italy). Nat Prod Res 2017, 31:2067-2071.

3. Arranz E, Jaime L, Lopez de las Hazas MC, et al. Supercritical fluid extraction as an alternative process to obtain essential oils with anti-inflammatory properties from marjoram and sweet basil. Industrial Crops and Products 2015, 67:121-129.

4. Bagamboula CF, Uyttendaele M, Debevere J. Inhibitory effect of thyme and basil essential oils, carvacrol, thymol, estragol, linalool and p-cymene towards Shigella sonnei and S. flexneri. Food Microbiology 2004, 21:33-42.

5. Elgayyar M, Draughon FA, Golden DA, Mount JR. Antimicrobial activity of essential oils from plants against selected pathogenic and saprophytic microorganisms. J Food Prot 2001, 64:1019-1024.

6. Hussain AI, Anwar F, Hussain Sherazi ST, Przybylski R. Chemical composition, antioxidant and antimicrobial activities of basil (Ocimum basilicum) essential oils depends on seasonal variations. Food Chem 2008, 108:986-995.

7. Muller GC, Junnila A, Butler J, et al. Efficacy of the botanical repellents geraniol, linalool, and citronella against mosquitoes. J Vector Ecol 2009, 34:2-8.

Bean sprouts

1. Guo X, Li T, Tang K, Liu RH. Effect of germination on phytochemical profiles and antioxidant activity of mung bean sprouts (Vigna radiata). J Agric Food Chem 2012, 60:11050-11055.

2. Devi CB, Kushwaha A, Kumar A. Sprouting characteristics and associated changes in nutritional composition of cowpea (Vigna unguiculata). J Food Sci Technol 2015, 52:6821-6827.

3. Fouad AA, Rehab FM. Effect of germination time on proximate analysis, bioactive compounds and antioxidant activity of lentil (Lens culinaris Medik.) sprouts. Acta Sci Pol Technol Aliment 2015, 14:233-246.

4. Hafidh RR, Abdulamir AS, Bakar FA, et al. Novel molecular, cytotoxical, and immunological study on promising and selective anticancer activity of mung bean sprouts. BMC Complement Altern Med 2012, 12:208.

Beans

1. Papanikolaou Y, Fulgoni VL, 3rd. Bean consumption is associated with greater nutrient intake, reduced systolic blood pressure, lower body weight, and a smaller waist circumference in adults: results from the National Health and Nutrition Examination Survey 1999-2002. J Am Coll Nutr 2008, 27:569-576.

2. Salehi-Abargouei A, Saraf-Bank S, Bellissimo N, Azadbakht L. Effects of non-soy legume consumption on C-reactive protein: a systematic review and meta-analysis. Nutrition 2015, 31:631-639.

3. Jayalath VH, de Souza RJ, Sievenpiper JL, et al. Effect of dietary pulses on blood pressure: a systematic review and meta-analysis of controlled feeding trials. Am J Hypertens 2014, 27:56-64.

4. Bazzano LA, Thompson AM, Tees MT, et al. Non-soy legume consumption lowers cholesterol levels: a meta-analysis of randomized controlled trials. Nutrition, metabolism, and cardiovascular diseases : NMCD 2011, 21:94-103.

5. Sievenpiper JL, Kendall CW, Esfahani A, et al. Effect of non-oil-seed pulses on glycaemic control: a systematic review and meta-analysis of randomised controlled experimental trials in people with and without diabetes. Diab tologia 2009, 52:1479-1495.

6. Zhu B, Sun Y, Qi L, et al. Dietary legume consumption reduces risk of colorectal cancer: evidence from a meta-analysis of cohort studies. Sci Rep 2015, 5:8797.

7. Li J, Mao QQ. Legume intake and risk of prostate cancer: a meta-analysis of prospective cohort studies. Oncotarget 2017, 8:44776-44784.

8. Aubertin-Leheudre M, Gorbach S, Woods M, et al. Fat/fiber intakes and sex hormones in healthy premenopausal women in USA. J Steroid Biochem Mol Biol 2008, 112:32-39.

9. Aubertin-Leheudre M, Hamalainen E, Adlercreutz H. Diets and hormonal levels in postmenopausal women with or without breast cancer. Nutr Cancer 2011, 63:514-524.

10. Goldin BR, Adlercreutz H, Gorbach SL, et al. Estrogen excretion patterns and plasma levels in vegetarian and omnivorous women. N Engl J Med 1982, 307:1542-1547.

11. Bernstein L, Ross RK. Endogenous hormones and breast cancer risk. Epidemiol Rev 1993, 15:48-65.

Beets
1. Dominguez R, Mate-Munoz JL, Cuenca E, et al. Effects of beetroot juice supplementation on intermittent high-intensity exercise efforts. J Int Soc Sports Nutr 2018, 15:2.

2. Dominguez R, Cuenca E, Mate-Munoz JL, et al. Effects of Beetroot Juice Supplementation on Cardiorespiratory Endurance in Athletes. A Systematic Review. Nutrients 2017, 9.

3. Clifford T, Howatson G, West DJ, Stevenson EJ. The potential benefits of red beetroot supplementation in health and disease. Nutrients 2015, 7:2801-2822.

Blackberries
1. Kaume L, Howard LR, Devareddy L. The Blackberry Fruit: A Review on Its Composition and Chemistry, Metabolism and Bioavailability, and Health Benefits. Journal of Agricultural and Food Chemistry 2011.

2. Aghababaee SK, Vafa M, Shidfar F, et al. Effects of blackberry (Morus nigra L.) consumption on serum concentration of lipoproteins, apo A-I, apo B, and high-sensitivity-C-reactive protein and blood pressure in dyslipidemic patients. J Res Med Sci 2015, 20:684-691.

Blueberries
1. Rocha D, Caldas A, da Silva B, et al. Effects of blueberry and cranberry consumption on type 2 diabetes glycemic control: a systematic review. Crit Rev Food Sci Nutr 2018:0.

2. Johnson SA, Figueroa A, Navaei N, et al. Daily blueberry consumption improves blood pressure and arterial stiffness in postmenopausal women with pre- and stage 1-hypertension: a randomized, double-blind, placebo-controlled clinical trial. J Acad Nutr Diet 2015, 115:369-377.

3. Cassidy A, O'Reilly EJ, Kay C, et al. Habitual intake of flavonoid subclasses and incident hypertension in adults. Am J Clin Nutr 2011, 93:338-347.

4. Bioactive Compounds in Berries Can Reduce High Blood Pressure. In ScienceDaily, 2011 [http://www.sciencedaily.com/releases/2011/01/110114155241.htm]

5. Krikorian R, Shidler MD, Nash TA, et al. Blueberry supplementation improves memory in older adults. Journal of agricultural and food chemistry 2010, 58:3996-4000.

6. Bowtell JL, Aboo-Bakkar Z, Conway M, et al. Enhanced task related brain activation and resting perfusion in healthy older adults after chronic blueberry supplementation. Appl Physiol Nutr Metab 2017.

7. Stoner GD, Wang LS, Casto BC. Laboratory and clinical studies of cancer chemoprevention by antioxidants in berries. Carcinogenesis 2008, 29:1665-1674.

8. Afrin S, Giampieri F, Gasparrini M, et al. Chemopreventive and Therapeutic Effects of Edible Berries: A Focus on Colon Cancer Prevention and Treatment. Molecules 2016, 21:169.

Bok Choy
1. Office of Dietary Supplements, Natinal Institutes of Health. Dietary Supplement Fact Sheet: Vitamin A. In 2016 [https://ods.od.nih.gov/factsheets/VitaminA-HealthProfessional/]

Broccoli
1. Bai Y, Wang X, Zhao S, et al. Sulforaphane Protects against Cardiovascular Disease via Nrf2 Activation. Oxid Med Cell Longev 2015, 2015:407580.

Broccoli Rabe
1.Zhang X, Shu XO, Xiang YB, et al. Cruciferous vegetable consumption is associated with a reduced risk of total and cardiovascular disease mortality. Am J Clin Nutr 2011, 94:240-246.

2. Pollock RL. The effect of green leafy and cruciferous vegetable intake on the incidence of cardiovascular disease: A meta-analysis. JRSM Cardiovasc Dis 2016, 5:2048004016661435.

3. Higdon J, Delage B, Williams D, Dashwood R. Cruciferous vegetables and human cancer risk: epidemiologic evidence and mechanistic basis. Pharmacol Res 2007, 55:224-236.

Brussels Sprouts
1. SNPedia: TASR238 [https://www.snpedia.com/index.php/TAS2R38]

2. Hoelzl C, Glatt H, Meinl W, et al. Consumption of Brussels sprouts protects peripheral human lymphocytes against 2-amino-1-methyl-6-phenylimidazo[4,5-b]pyridine (PhIP) and oxidative DNA-damage: results of a controlled human intervention trial. Mol Nutr Food Res 2008, 52:330-341.

Cabbage (Red, Nappa)
1. Higdon J, Drake VJ, Delage B. Linus Pauling Institute, Oregon State University. Micronutrient Information Center. Cruciferous Vegetables. In 2016 [http://lpi.oregonstate.edu/mic/food-beverages/cruciferous-vegetables]

2. Liu B, Mao Q, Lin Y, et al. The association of cruciferous vegetables intake and risk of bladder cancer: a meta-analysis. World J Urol 2012.

3. Liu B, Mao Q, Cao M, Xie L. Cruciferous vegetables intake and risk of prostate cancer: a meta-analysis. Int J Urol 2012, 19:134-141.

4. Hu J, Hu Y, Hu Y, Zheng S. Intake of cruciferous vegetables is associated with reduced risk of ovarian cancer: a meta-analysis. Asia Pac J Clin Nutr 2015, 24:101-109.

5. Wu QJ, Yang Y, Wang J, et al. Cruciferous vegetable consumption and gastric cancer risk: a meta-analysis of epidemiological studies. Cancer Sci 2013, 104:1067-1073.

6. Wu QJ, Yang Y, Vogtmann E, et al. Cruciferous vegetables intake and the risk of colorectal cancer: a meta-analysis of observational studies. Ann Oncol 2013, 24:1079-1087.

7. Wu QJ, Xie L, Zheng W, et al. Cruciferous vegetables consumption and the risk of female lung cancer: a prospective study and a meta-analysis. Ann Oncol 2013, 24:1918-1924.

Carrots

1. Shardell MD, Alley DE, Hicks GE, et al. Low-serum carotenoid concentrations and carotenoid interactions predict mortality in US adults: the Third National Health and Nutrition Examination Survey. Nutr Res 2011, 31:178-189.

2. Min KB, Min JY. Association between leukocyte telomere length and serum carotenoid in US adults. Eur J Nutr 2016.

3. Oregon State University. Linus Pauling Institute Micronutrient Information Center. Vitamin A. In [http://lpi.oregonstate.edu/infocenter/vitamins/vitaminA/]

4. Kobaek-Larsen M, El-Houri RB, Christensen LP, et al. Dietary polyacetylenes, falcarinol and falcarindiol, isolated from carrots prevents the formation of neoplastic lesions in the colon of azoxymethane-induced rats. Food Funct 2017, 8:964-974.

5. van Het Hof KH, West CE, Weststrate JA, Hautvast JG. Dietary factors that affect the bioavailability of carotenoids. J Nutr 2000, 130:503-506.

6. Talcott ST, Howard LR, Brenes CH. Antioxidant changes and sensory properties of carrot puree processed with and without periderm tissue. J Agric Food Chem 2000, 48:1315-1321.

7. Brown MJ, Ferruzzi MG, Nguyen ML, et al. Carotenoid bioavailability is higher from salads ingested with full-fat than with fat-reduced salad dressings as measured with electrochemical detection. Am J Clin Nutr 2004, 80:396-403.

Cashews

1. Kris-Etherton PM. Walnuts decrease risk of cardiovascular disease: a summary of efficacy and biologic mechanisms. J Nutr 2014, 144:547S-554S.

2. Grosso G, Yang J, Marventano S, et al. Nut consumption on all-cause, cardiovascular, and cancer mortality risk: a systematic review and meta-analysis of epidemiologic studies. Am J Clin Nutr 2015, 101:783-793.

3. Ma Y, Njike VY, Millet J, et al. Effects of walnut consumption

on endothelial function in type 2 diabetic subjects: a randomized controlled crossover trial. Diabetes Care 2010, 33:227-232.

4. Mattes RD, Dreher ML. Nuts and healthy body weight maintenance mechanisms. Asia Pac J Clin Nutr 2010, 19:137-141.

5. Mohan V, Gayathri R, Jaacks LM, et al. Cashew Nut Consumption Increases HDL Cholesterol and Reduces Systolic Blood Pressure in Asian Indians with Type 2 Diabetes: A 12-Week Randomized Controlled Trial. J Nutr 2018, 148:63-69.

6. Mah E, Schulz JA, Kaden VN, et al. Cashew consumption reduces total and LDL cholesterol: a randomized, crossover, controlled-feeding trial. Am J Clin Nutr 2017, 105:1070-1078.

Cauliflower

1. Hanschen FS, Schreiner M. Isothiocyanates, Nitriles, and Epithionitriles from Glucosinolates Are Affected by Genotype and Developmental Stage in Brassica oleracea Varieties. Front Plant Sci 2017, 8:1095.

2. Liu B, Mao Q, Lin Y, et al. The association of cruciferous vegetables intake and risk of bladder cancer: a meta-analysis. World J Urol 2012.

3. Liu B, Mao Q, Cao M, Xie L. Cruciferous vegetables intake and risk of prostate cancer: a meta-analysis. Int J Urol 2012, 19:134-141.

4. Hu J, Hu Y, Hu Y, Zheng S. Intake of cruciferous vegetables is associated with reduced risk of ovarian cancer: a meta-analysis. Asia Pac J Clin Nutr 2015, 24:101-109.

5. Wu QJ, Yang Y, Wang J, et al. Cruciferous vegetable consumption and gastric cancer risk: a meta-analysis of epidemiological studies. Cancer Sci 2013, 104:1067-1073.

6. Wu QJ, Yang Y, Vogtmann E, et al. Cruciferous vegetables intake and the risk of colorectal cancer: a meta-analysis of observational studies. Ann Oncol 2013, 24:1079-1087.

7. Wu QJ, Xie L, Zheng W, et al. Cruciferous vegetables consumption and the risk of female lung cancer: a prospective study and a meta-analysis. Ann Oncol 2013, 24:1918-1924.

8. Shaw GM, Carmichael SL, Yang W, et al. Periconceptional dietary intake of choline and betaine and neural tube defects in offspring. Am J Epidemiol 2004, 160:102-109.

9. Zeisel SH. Nutrition in pregnancy: the argument for including a source of choline. Int J Womens Health 2013, 5:193-199.

10. Boeke CE, Gillman MW, Hughes MD, et al. Choline intake during pregnancy and child cognition at age 7 years. Am J Epidemiol 2013, 177:1338-1347.

Cherries

1. Connolly DA, McHugh MP, Padilla-Zakour OI, et al. Efficacy of a tart cherry juice blend in preventing the symptoms of muscle damage. Br J Sports Med 2006, 40:679-683; discussion 683.

2. Kuehl KS, Perrier ET, Elliot DL, Chesnutt JC. Efficacy of tart

cherry juice in reducing muscle pain during running: a randomized controlled trial. J Int Soc Sports Nutr 2010, 7:17.

3. Levers K, Dalton R, Galvan E, et al. Effects of powdered Montmorency tart cherry supplementation on acute endurance exercise performance in aerobically trained individuals. J Int Soc Sports Nutr 2016, 13:22.

4. Levers K, Dalton R, Galvan E, et al. Effects of powdered Montmorency tart cherry supplementation on an acute bout of intense lower body strength exercise in resistance trained males. J Int Soc Sports Nutr 2015, 12:41.

5. Martin KR, Bopp J, Burrell L, Hook G: The effect of 100% tart cherry juice on serum uric acid levels, biomarkers of inflammation and cardiovascular disease risk factors. In Experimental Biology 2011. Washington, D.C.: The Federation of American Societies for Experimental Biology; 2011.

6. Kelley DS, Rasooly R, Jacob RA, et al. Consumption of Bing sweet cherries lowers circulating concentrations of inflammation markers in healthy men and women. J Nutr 2006, 136:981-986.

7. Keane KM, George TW, Constantinou CL, et al. Effects of Montmorency tart cherry (Prunus Cerasus L.) consumption on vascular function in men with early hypertension. Am J Clin Nutr 2016, 103:1531-1539.

8. Jacob RA, Spinozzi GM, Simon VA, et al. Consumption of cherries lowers plasma urate in healthy women. J Nutr 2003, 133:1826-1829.

9. Ferretti G, Bacchetti T, Belleggia A, Neri D. Cherry antioxidants: from farm to table. Molecules 2010, 15:6993-7005.

10. Traustadottir T, Davies SS, Stock AA, et al. Tart cherry juice decreases oxidative stress in healthy older men and women. J Nutr 2009, 139:1896-1900.

11. Burkhardt S, Tan DX, Manchester LC, et al. Detection and quantification of the antioxidant melatonin in Montmorency and Balaton tart cherries (Prunus cerasus). J Agric Food Chem 2001, 49:4898-4902.

12. Pigeon WR, Carr M, Gorman C, Perlis ML. Effects of a tart cherry juice beverage on the sleep of older adults with insomnia: a pilot study. J Med Food 2010, 13:579-583.

Chia Seeds

1. USDA National Nutrient Database for Standard Reference [http://ndb.nal.usda.gov/ndb/search/list]

2. Vuksan V, Whitham D, Sievenpiper JL, et al. Supplementation of conventional therapy with the novel grain Salba (Salvia hispanica L.) improves major and emerging cardiovascular risk factors in type 2 diabetes: results of a randomized controlled trial. Diabetes Care 2007, 30:2804-2810.

3. Toscano LT, da Silva CS, Toscano LT, et al. Chia flour supplementation reduces blood pressure in hypertensive subjects. Plant Foods Hum Nutr 2014, 69:392-398.

4. Vuksan V, Jenkins AL, Brissette C, et al. Salba-chia (Salvia hispanica L.) in the treatment of overweight and obese patients with type 2 diabetes: A double-blind randomized controlled trial. Nutr Metab Cardiovasc Dis 2017, 27:138-146.

5. Nemes SM, Orstat V. Evaluation of a Microwave-Assisted Extraction Method for Lignan Quantification in Flaxseed Cultivars and Selected Oil Seeds. Food Analytical Methods 2012, 5:551-563.

6. Azrad M, Vollmer RT, Madden J, et al. Flaxseed-derived enterolactone is inversely associated with tumor cell proliferation in men with localized prostate cancer. J Med Food 2013, 16:357-360.

7. Buck K, Zaineddin AK, Vrieling A, et al. Meta-analyses of lignans and enterolignans in relation to breast cancer risk. Am J Clin Nutr 2010, 92:141-153.

Cinnamon

1. Abraham K, Wohrlin F, Lindtner O, et al. Toxicology and risk assessment of coumarin: focus on human data. Mol Nutr Food Res 2010, 54:228-239.

2. Fotland TO, Paulsen JE, Sanner T, et al. Risk assessment of coumarin using the bench mark dose (BMD) approach: children in Norway which regularly eat oatmeal porridge with cinnamon may exceed the TDI for coumarin with several folds. Food Chem Toxicol 2012, 50:903-912.

3. Blahova J, Svobodova Z. Assessment of coumarin levels in ground cinnamon available in the Czech retail market. ScientificWorldJournal 2012, 2012:263851.

4. Gunawardena D, Karunaweera N, Lee S, et al. Anti-inflammatory activity of cinnamon (C. zeylanicum and C. cassia) extracts - identification of E-cinnamaldehyde and o-methoxy cinnamaldehyde as the most potent bioactive compounds. Food Funct 2015, 6:910-919.

5. Lee SH, Lee SY, Son DJ, et al. Inhibitory effect of 2'-hydroxy-cinnamaldehyde on nitric oxide production through inhibition of NF-kappa B activation in RAW 264.7 cells. Biochem Pharmacol 2005, 69:791-799.

6. Davis PA, Yokoyama W. Cinnamon intake lowers fasting blood glucose: meta-analysis. J Med Food 2011; 14:884-889.

Cacao powder/cocoa powder

1. Desch S, Schmidt J, Kobler D, et al. Effect of cocoa products on blood pressure: systematic review and meta-analysis. Am J Hypertens 2010, 23:97-103.

2. Ried K, Sullivan TR, Fakler P, et al. Effect of cocoa on blood pressure. Cochrane Database Syst Rev 2012, 8:CD008893.

3. Aprotosoaie AC, Miron A, Trifan A, et al. The Cardiovascular Effects of Cocoa Polyphenols-An Overview. Diseases 2016, 4.

4. Lin X, Zhang I, Li A, et al. Cocoa Flavanol Intake and Biomarkers for Cardiometabolic Health: A Systematic Review and

Meta-Analysis of Randomized Controlled Trials. J Nutr 2016, 146:2325-2333.

5. Socci V, Tempesta D, Desideri G, et al. Enhancing Human Cognition with Cocoa Flavonoids. Front Nutr 2017, 4:19.

Collards

1. Higdon J, Delage B, Williams D, Dashwood R. Cruciferous vegetables and human cancer risk: epidemiologic evidence and mechanistic basis. Pharmacol Res 2007, 55:224-236.

2. Liu B, Mao Q, Lin Y, et al. The association of cruciferous vegetables intake and risk of bladder cancer: a meta-analysis. World J Urol 2012.

3. Liu B, Mao Q, Cao M, Xie L. Cruciferous vegetables intake and risk of prostate cancer: a meta-analysis. Int J Urol 2012, 19:134-141.

4. Hu J, Hu Y, Hu Y, Zheng S. Intake of cruciferous vegetables is associated with reduced risk of ovarian cancer: a meta-analysis. Asia Pac J Clin Nutr 2015, 24:101-109.

5. Wu QJ, Yang Y, Wang J, et al. Cruciferous vegetable consumption and gastric cancer risk: a meta-analysis of epidemiological studies. Cancer Sci 2013, 104:1067-1073.

6. Wu QJ, Yang Y, Vogtmann E, et al. Cruciferous vegetables intake and the risk of colorectal cancer: a meta-analysis of observational studies. Ann Oncol 2013, 24:1079-1087.

7. Wu QJ, Xie L, Zheng W, et al. Cruciferous vegetables consumption and the risk of female lung cancer: a prospective study and a meta-analysis. Ann Oncol 2013, 24:1918-1924.

8. Zhang X, Shu XO, Xiang YB, Yang G, Li H, Gao J, Cai H, Gao YT, Zheng W. Cruciferous vegetable consumption is associated with a reduced risk of total and cardiovascular disease mortality. Am J Clin Nutr 2011; 94:240-246.

Corn

1. Srinivasan M, Sudheer AR, Menon VP. Ferulic Acid: therapeutic potential through its antioxidant property. J Clin Biochem Nutr 2007, 40:92-100.

2. Dewanto V, Wu X, Liu RH. Processed sweet corn has higher antioxidant activity. J Agric Food Chem 2002, 50:4959-4964.

3. Bednar GE, Patil AR, Murray SM, et al. Starch and fiber fractions in selected food and feed ingredients affect their small intestinal digestibility and fermentability and their large bowel fermentability in vitro in a canine model. J Nutr 2001, 131:276-286.

4. Hamer HM, Jonkers D, Venema K, et al. Review article: the role of butyrate on colonic function. Aliment Pharmacol Ther 2008, 27:104-119.

5. Guyton KZ, Loomis D, Grosse Y, et al. Carcinogenicity of tetrachlorvinphos, parathion, malathion, diazinon, and glyphosate. Lancet Oncol 2015, 16:490-491.

6. Rojano-Delgado AM, Ruiz-Jimenez J, de Castro MD, De Prado R. Determination of glyphosate and its metabolites in plant material by reversed-polarity CE with indirect absorptiometric detection. Electophoresis 2010, 31:1423-1430.

Cranberries

1. Wang CH, Fang CC, Chen NC, et al. Cranberry-Containing Products for Prevention of Urinary Tract Infections in Susceptible Populations: A Systematic Review and Meta-analysis of Randomized Controlled Trials. Arch Intern Med 2012, 172:988-996.

2. Blumberg JB, Camesano TA, Cassidy A, et al. Cranberries and their bioactive constituents in human health. Adv Nutr 2013, 4:618-632.

3. Paquette M, Medina Larque AS, Weisnagel SJ, et al. Strawberry and cranberry polyphenols improve insulin sensitivity in insulin-resistant, non-diabetic adults: a parallel, double-blind, controlled and randomised clinical trial. Br J Nutr 2017, 117:519-531.

4. Dohadwala MM, Holbrook M, Hamburg NM, et al. Effects of cranberry juice consumption on vascular function in patients with coronary artery disease. Am J Clin Nutr 2011.

Cucumber

1. Min KJ, Nam JO, Kwon TK. Fisetin Induces Apoptosis Through p53-Mediated Up-Regulation of DR5 Expression in Human Renal Carcinoma Caki Cells. Molecules 2017, 22.

2. Ahmad A, Ali T, Park HY, et al. Neuroprotective Effect of Fisetin Against Amyloid-Beta-Induced Cognitive/Synaptic Dysfunction, Neuroinflammation, and Neurodegeneration in Adult Mice. Mol Neurobiol 2017, 54:2269-2285.

3. Singh S, Singh AK, Garg G, Rizvi SI. Fisetin as a caloric restriction mimetic protects rat brain against aging induced oxidative stress, apoptosis and neurodegeneration. Life Sci 2017.

Dill

1. Carlsen MH, Halvorsen BL, Holte K, et al. The total antioxidant content of more than 3100 foods, beverages, spices, herbs and supplements used worldwide. Nutrition Journal 2010, 9:3.

2. Kaefer CM, Milner JA: Herbs and Spices in Cancer Prevention and Treatment. In Herbal Medicine: Biomolecular and Clinical Aspects. Edited by Benzie IFF, Wachtel-Galor S. Boca Raton (FL)2011

3. Spices May Protect Against Consequences Of High Blood Sugar. In ScienceDaily, 2008. https://www.sciencedaily.com/releases/2008/08/080805153830.htm

4. Tian J, Ban X, Zeng H, et al. The mechanism of antifungal action of essential oil from dill (Anethum graveolens L.) on Aspergillus flavus. PLoS One 2012, 7:e30147.

Edamame

1. Messina M. Soy foods, isoflavones, and the health of postmenopausal women. Am J Clin Nutr 2014, 100 Suppl 1:423S-430S.

2. Messina M. Insights gained from 20 years of soy research. J Nutr 2010, 140:2289S-2295S.

3. Hwang YW, Kim SY, Jee SH, et al. Soy food consumption and risk of prostate cancer: a meta-analysis of observational studies. Nutr Cancer 2009, 61:598-606.

4. Yang WS, Va P, Wong MY, et al. Soy intake is associated with lower lung cancer risk: results from a meta-analysis of epidemiologic studies. Am J Clin Nutr 2011, 94:1575-1583.

5. Kim J, Kang M, Lee JS, et al. Fermented and non-fermented soy food consumption and gastric cancer in Japanese and Korean populations: a meta-analysis of observational studies. Cancer Sci 2011, 102:231-244.

6.Y an L, Spitznagel EL, Bosland MC. Soy consumption and colorectal cancer risk in humans: a meta-analysis. Cancer Epidemiol Biomarkers Prev 2010, 19:148-158.

7. Oseni T, Patel R, Pyle J, Jordan VC. Selective estrogen receptor modulators and phytoestrogens. Planta Med 2008, 74:1656-1665.

Eggplant

1. Komatsu W, Itoh K, Akutsu S, et al. Nasunin inhibits the lipopolysaccharide-induced pro-inflammatory mediator production in RAW264 mouse macrophages by suppressing ROS-mediated activation of PI3 K/Akt/NF-kappaB and p38 signaling pathways. Biosci Biotechnol Biochem 2017, 81:1956-1966.

2. Matsubara K, Kaneyuki T, Miyake T, Mori M. Antiangiogenic activity of nasunin, an antioxidant anthocyanin, in eggplant peels. J Agric Food Chem 2005, 53:6272-6275.

3. Noda Y, Kneyuki T, Igarashi K, et al. Antioxidant activity of nasunin, an anthocyanin in eggplant peels. Toxicology 2000, 148:119-123.

Endive

1. Chen AY, Chen YC. A review of the dietary flavonoid, kaempferol on human health and cancer chemoprevention. Food Chem 2013, 138:2099-2107.

2. Hua X, Yu L, You R, et al. Association among Dietary Flavonoids, Flavonoid Subclasses and Ovarian Cancer Risk: A Meta-Analysis. PLoS One 2016, 11:e0151134.

3. Xie Y, Huang S, Su Y. Dietary Flavonols Intake and Risk of Esophageal and Gastric Cancer: A Meta-Analysis of Epidemiological Studies. Nutrients 2016, 8:91.

4. Hui C, Qi X, Qianyong Z, et al. Flavonoids, flavonoid subclasses and breast cancer risk: a meta-analysis of epidemiologic studies. PLoS One 2013, 8:e54318.

Escarole

1. Zhang S, Won YK, Ong CN, Shen HM. Anti-cancer potential of sesquiterpene lactones: bioactivity and molecular mechanisms. Curr Med Chem Anticancer Agents 2005; 5:239-249.

2. Woyengo TA, Ramprasath VR, Jones PJ. Anticancer effects of phytosterols. Eur J Clin Nutr 2009; 63:813-820.

Fennel

1. Picon PD, Picon RV, Costa AF, et al. Randomized clinical trial of a phytotherapic compound containing Pimpinella anisum, Foeniculum vulgare, Sambucus nigra, and Cassia augustifolia for chronic constipation. BMC Complement Altern Med 2010, 10:17.

2. Rahimikian F, Rahimi R, Golzareh P, et al. Effect of Foeniculum vulgare Mill. (fennel) on menopausal symptoms in post-menopausal women: a randomized, triple-blind, placebo-controlled trial. Menopause 2017.

3. Chainy GB, Manna SK, Chaturvedi MM, Aggarwal BB. Anethole blocks both early and late cellular responses transduced by tumor necrosis factor: effect on NF-kappaB, AP-1, JNK, MAPKK and apoptosis. Oncogene 2000, 19:2943-2950.

4. Sung B, Prasad S, Yadav VR, Aggarwal BB. Cancer cell signaling pathways targeted by spice-derived nutraceuticals. Nutr Cancer 2012, 64:173-197.

Figs

1. California Figs: Nutrition [http://californiafigs.com/nutrition.php]

2. Streppel MT, Arends LR, van 't Veer P, et al. Dietary fiber and blood pressure: a meta-analysis of randomized placebo-controlled trials. Arch Intern Med 2005, 165:150-156.

3. Brown L, Rosner B, Willett WW, Sacks FM. Cholesterol-lowering effects of dietary fiber: a meta-analysis. Am J Clin Nutr 1999, 69:30-42.

4. Higdon J, Drake VJ: Fiber. In An Evidence-based Approach to Phytochemicals and Other Dietary Factors New York: Thieme; 2013: 133-148

5. Ercisli S, Tosun M, Karlidag H, et al. Color and antioxidant characteristics of some fresh fig (Ficus carica L.) genotypes from northeastern Turkey. Plant Foods Hum Nutr 2012, 67:271-276.

6. Vinson JA, Zubik L, Bose P, et al. Dried fruits: excellent in vitro and in vivo antioxidants. J Am Coll Nutr 2005, 24:44-50.

7. Serraclara A, Hawkins F, Perez C, et al. Hypoglycemic action of an oral fig-leaf decoction in type-I diabetic patients. Diabetes Res Clin Pract 1998, 39:19-22.

Flax seeds

1. Khalesi S, Irwin C, Schubert M. Flaxseed consumption may reduce blood pressure: a systematic review and meta-analysis of controlled trials. J Nutr 2015, 145:758-765.

2. Sturgeon SR, Heersink JL, Volpe SL, et al. Effect of dietary flaxseed on serum levels of estrogens and androgens in post-menopausal women. Nutr Cancer 2008, 60:612-618.

3. Buck K, Zaineddin AK, Vrieling A, et al. Meta-analyses of lignans and enterolignans in relation to breast cancer risk. Am J Clin Nutr 2010, 92:141-153.

4. Adlercreutz H. Lignans and human health. Crit Rev Clin Lab Sci 2007, 44:483-525.

5. Thompson LU, Chen JM, Li T, et al. Dietary flaxseed alters tumor biological markers in postmenopausal breast cancer. Clin Cancer Res 2005, 11:3828-3835.

Garlic

1. Arreola R, Quintero-Fabian S, Lopez-Roa RI, et al. Immunomodulation and anti-inflammatory effects of garlic compounds. J Immunol Res 2015, 2015:401630.

2. Powolny A, Singh S. Multitargeted prevention and therapy of cancer by diallyl trisulfide and related Allium vegetable-derived organosulfur compounds. Cancer Lett 2008, 269:305-314.

3. Rahman K, Lowe GM. Garlic and cardiovascular disease: a critical review. J Nutr 2006, 136:736S-740S.

4. Bradley JM, Organ CL, Lefer DJ. Garlic-Derived Organic Polysulfides and Myocardial Protection. J Nutr 2016, 146:403S-409S.

5. Galeone C, Pelucchi C, Levi F, et al. Onion and garlic use and human cancer. Am J Clin Nutr 2006, 84:1027-1032.

Ginger

1. Prasad S, Tyagi AK. Ginger and its constituents: role in prevention and treatment of gastrointestinal cancer. Gastroenterol Res Pract 2015, 2015:142979.

2. Kaur IP, Deol PK, Kondepudi KK, Bishnoi M. Anticancer Potential of Ginger: Mechanistic and Pharmacological Aspects. Curr Pharm Des 2016, 22:4160-4172.

3. Kim EC, Min JK, Kim TY, et al. [6]-Gingerol, a pungent ingredient of ginger, inhibits angiogenesis in vitro and in vivo. Biochem Biophys Res Commun 2005, 335:300-308.

4. White B. Ginger: an overview. Am Fam Physician 2007, 75:1689-1691.

5. Bartels EM, Folmer VN, Bliddal H, et al. Efficacy and safety of ginger in osteoarthritis patients: a meta-analysis of randomized placebo-controlled trials. Osteoarthritis Cartilage 2015, 23:13-21.

6. Maghbooli M, Golipour F, Moghimi Esfandabadi A, Yousefi M. Comparison between the efficacy of ginger and sumatriptan in the ablative treatment of the common migraine. Phytother Res 2014, 28:412-415.

7. Chen CX, Barrett B, Kwekkeboom KL. Efficacy of Oral Ginger (Zingiber officinale) for Dysmenorrhea: A Systematic Review and Meta-Analysis. Evid Based Complement Alternat Med 2016, 2016:6295737.

8. Daily JW, Zhang X, Kim DS, Park S. Efficacy of Ginger for Alleviating the Symptoms of Primary Dysmenorrhea: A Systematic Review and Meta-analysis of Randomized Clinical Trials. Pain Med 2015, 16:2243-2255.

Goji Berries

1. Widomska J, Subczynski WK. Why has Nature Chosen Lutein and Zeaxanthin to Protect the Retina? J Clin Exp Ophthalmol 2014, 5:326.

2. Gao Y, Wei Y, Wang Y, et al. Lycium Barbarum: A Traditional Chinese Herb and A Promising Anti-Aging Agent. Aging Dis 2017, 8:778-791.

3. Cheng J, Zhou ZW, Sheng HP, et al. An evidence-based update on the pharmacological activities and possible molecular targets of Lycium barbarum polysaccharides. Drug Des Devel Ther 2015, 9:33-78.

Gooseberries

1. Zhao T, Sun Q, Marques M, Witcher M. Anticancer Properties of Phyllanthus emblica (Indian Gooseberry). Oxid Med Cell Longev 2015, 2015:950890.

2. Akhtar MS, Ramzan A, Ali A, Ahmad M. Effect of Amla fruit (Emblica officinalis Gaertn.) on blood glucose and lipid profile of normal subjects and type 2 diabetic patients. Int J Food Sci Nutr 2011, 62:609-616.

3. Jacob A, Pandey M, Kapoor S, Saroja R. Effect of the Indian gooseberry (amla) on serum cholesterol levels in men aged 35-55 years. Eur J Clin Nutr 1988, 42:939-944.

Grains (Steel-Cut Oats, Barley, Teff, Buckwheat)

1. Higdon J, Drake VJ: Fiber. In An Evidence-based Approach to Phytochemicals and Other Dietary Factors New York: Thieme; 2013:133-148

2. Aune D, Chan DS, Lau R, et al. Dietary fibre, whole grains, and risk of colorectal cancer: systematic review and dose-response meta-analysis of prospective studies. BMJ 2011, 343:d6617.

3. Brown L, Rosner B, Willett WW, Sacks FM. Cholesterol-lowering effects of dietary fiber: a meta-analysis. Am J Clin Nutr 1999, 69:30-42.

4. Kreft M. Buckwheat phenolic metabolites in health and disease. Nutr Res Rev 2016, 29:30-39.

5. Ghorbani A. Mechanisms of antidiabetic effects of flavonoid rutin. Biomed Pharmacother 2017, 96:305-312.

Grapes

1. Rahbar AR, Mahmoudabadi MM, Islam MS: Comparative effects of red and white grapes on oxidative markers and lipidemic parameters in adult hypercholesterolemic humans. Food Funct 2015;6:1992-1998.

2. Barona J, Blesso CN, Andersen CJ, et al: Grape consumption increases anti-inflammatory markers and upregulates peripheral nitric oxide synthase in the absence of dyslipidemias in men with metabolic syndrome. Nutrients 2012;4:1945-1957.

3. Nguyen AV, Martinez M, Stamos MJ, et al: Results of a phase I

pilot clinical trial examining the effect of plant-derived resveratrol and grape powder on Wnt pathway target gene expression in colonic mucosa and colon cancer. Cancer Manag Res 2009;1:25-37.

Green beans

1. Oregon State University. Linus Pauling Institute. Micronutrient Information Center: Vitamin K [http://lpi.oregonstate.edu/infocenter/vitamins/vitamink/]

2. Jugdaohsingh R. Silicon and bone health. J Nutr Health Aging 2007; 11:99-110.

Green tea

1. Lorenz M, Stangl K, Stangl V. Vascular effects of tea are suppressed by soy milk. Atherosclerosis 2009, 206:31-32.

2. Lorenz M, Jochmann N, von Krosigk A, et al. Addition of milk prevents vascular protective effects of tea. Eur Heart J 2007, 28:219-223.

3. Wang ZM, Zhou B, Wang YS, et al. Black and green tea consumption and the risk of coronary artery disease: a meta-analysis. The American journal of clinical nutrition 2011, 93:506-515.

4. Arab L, Liu W, Elashoff D. Green and black tea consumption and risk of stroke: a meta-analysis. Stroke 2009, 40:1786-1792.

5. Tang N, Wu Y, Zhou B, et al. Green tea, black tea consumption and risk of lung cancer: a meta-analysis. Lung Cancer 2009, 65:274-283.

6. Sun CL, Yuan JM, Koh WP, Yu MC. Green tea, black tea and breast cancer risk: a meta-analysis of epidemiological studies. Carcinogenesis 2006, 27:1310-1315.

7. Ogunleye AA, Xue F, Michels KB. Green tea consumption and breast cancer risk or recurrence: a meta-analysis. Breast Cancer Res Treat 2010, 119:477-484.

8. Khan N, Adhami VM, Mukhtar H. Review: green tea polyphenols in chemoprevention of prostate cancer: preclinical and clinical studies. Nutr Cancer 2009, 61:836-841.

9. Zheng J, Yang B, Huang T, et al. Green Tea and Black Tea Consumption and Prostate Cancer Risk: An Exploratory Meta-Analysis of Observational Studies. Nutr Cancer 2011:1-10.

10. Kuriyama S, Shimazu T, Ohmori K, et al. Green tea consumption and mortality due to cardiovascular disease, cancer, and all causes in Japan: the Ohsaki study. JAMA 2006, 296:1255-1265.

11. Iso H, Date C, Wakai K, et al. The relationship between green tea and total caffeine intake and risk for self-reported type 2 diabetes among Japanese adults. Ann Intern Med 2006, 144:554-562.

12. Assuncao M, Andrade JP. Protective action of green tea catechins in neuronal mitochondria during aging. Front Biosci (Landmark Ed) 2015, 20:247-262.

13. Mandel SA, Amit T, Weinreb O, Youdim MB. Understanding the broad-spectrum neuroprotective action profile of green tea polyphenols in aging and neurodegenerative diseases. J Alzheimers Dis 2011, 25:187-208.

14. USDA Database for the Flavonoid Content of Selected Foods, Release 3 (2011) [http://www.ars.usda.gov/Services/docs.htm?docid=6231]

15. Astill C, Birch MR, Dacombe C, et al. Factors affecting the caffeine and polyphenol contents of black and green tea infusions. J Agric Food Chem 2001, 49:5340-5347.

16. Venditti E, Bacchetti T, Tiano L, et al. Hot vs. cold water steeping of different teas: Do they affect antioxidant activity? Food Chemistry 2010, 119:1597-1604.

Hazelnuts

1. Tey SL, Delahunty C, Gray A, et al. Effects of regular consumption of different forms of almonds and hazelnuts on acceptance and blood lipids. Eur J Nutr 2015, 54:483-487.

2. Tey SL, Brown RC, Chisholm AW, et al. Effects of different forms of hazelnuts on blood lipids and alpha-tocopherol concentrations in mildly hypercholesterolemic individuals. Eur J Clin Nutr 2011, 65:117-124.

3. Bolling BW, Chen CY, McKay DL, Blumberg JB. Tree nut phytochemicals: composition, antioxidant capacity, bioactivity, impact factors. A systematic review of almonds, Brazils, cashews, hazelnuts, macadamias, pecans, pine nuts, pistachios and walnuts. Nutr Res Rev 2011:1-32.

4. Di Renzo L, Merra G, Botta R, et al. Post-prandial effects of hazelnut-enriched high fat meal on LDL oxidative status, oxidative and inflammatory gene expression of healthy subjects: a randomized trial. Eur Rev Med Pharmacol Sci 2017, 21:1610-1626.

Hemp Seeds

1. Higdon J, Drake VJ: Essential Fatty Acids. In An Evidence-Based Approach to Dietary Phytochemicals and Other Dietary Factors. Second edition. New York: Thieme; 2013: 183-208

2. Montserrat-de la Paz S, Marin-Aguilar F, Garcia-Gimenez MD, Fernandez-Arche MA. Hemp (Cannabis sativa L.) seed oil: analytical and phytochemical characterization of the unsaponifiable fraction. J Agric Food Chem 2014, 62:1105-1110.

3. Callaway JC. Hempseed as a nutritional resource: An overview. Euphytica 2004, 140:65-72.

4. Industrial Hemp Production 2015 [https://www.uky.edu/Ag/CCD/introsheets/hempproduction.pdf]

Jackfruit

1. Liu B, Bian HJ, Bao JK. Plant lectins: potential antineoplastic drugs from bench to clinic. Cancer Lett 2010, 287:1-12.

2. Yu LG, Packman LC, Weldon M, et al. Protein phosphatase 2A, a negative regulator of the ERK signaling pathway, is activated by tyrosine phosphorylation of putative HLA class II-

144　　　　　　　　　　　　　　　　　　**100 Best Foods**

associated protein I (PHAPI)/pp32 in response to the antiproliferative lectin, jacalin. J Biol Chem 2004, 279:41377-41383.

3. Geraldino TH, Modiano P, Veronez LC, et al. Jacalin Has Chemopreventive Effects on Colon Cancer Development. Biomed Res Int 2017, 2017:4614357.

Kale

1. Higdon J, Drake VJ, Delage B: Linus Pauling Institute, Oregon State University. Micronutrient Information Center. Cruciferous Vegetables. 2016. http://lpi.oregonstate.edu/mic/food-beverages/cruciferous-vegetables. Accessed January 2018.

2. Higdon J, Delage B, Williams D, et al: Cruciferous vegetables and human cancer risk: epidemiologic evidence and mechanistic basis. Pharmacol Res 2007;55:224-236.

3. Zhang X, Shu XO, Xiang YB, et al: Cruciferous vegetable consumption is associated with a reduced risk of total and cardiovascular disease mortality. Am J Clin Nutr 2011;94:240-246.

4. Weaver CM, Plawecki KL: Dietary calcium: adequacy of a vegetarian diet. Am J Clin Nutr 1994;59:1238S-1241S.

Kiwi

1. Skinner MA, Loh JM, Hunter DC, Zhang J. Gold kiwifruit (Actinidia chinensis 'Hort16A') for immune support. Proc Nutr Soc 2011, 70:276-280.

2. Brevik A, Gaivao I, Medin T, et al. Supplementation of a western diet with golden kiwifruits (Actinidia chinensis var.'Hort 16A':) effects on biomarkers of oxidation damage and antioxidant protection. Nutr J 2011, 10:54.

3. Lin HH, Tsai PS, Fang SC, Liu JF. Effect of kiwifruit consumption on sleep quality in adults with sleep problems. Asia Pac J Clin Nutr 2011, 20:169-174.

4. Chang CC, Lin YT, Lu YT, et al. Kiwifruit improves bowel function in patients with irritable bowel syndrome with constipation. Asia Pac J Clin Nutr 2010, 19:451-457.

Kohlrabi

1. USDA National Nutrient Database for Standard Reference [http://ndb.nal.usda.gov/ndb/search/list]

2. Jung HA, Karki S, Ehom NY, et al. Anti-Diabetic and Anti-Inflammatory Effects of Green and Red Kohlrabi Cultivars (Brassica oleracea var. gongylodes). Prev Nutr Food Sci 2014, 19:281-290.

Kumquats

1. Sadek ES, Makris DP, Kefalas P. Polyphenolic composition and antioxidant characteristics of kumquat (Fortunella margarita) peel fractions. Plant Foods Hum Nutr 2009, 64:297-302.

2. Jayaprakasha GK, Murthy KN, Demarais R, Patil BS. Inhibition of prostate cancer (LNCaP) cell proliferation by volatile components from Nagami kumquats. Planta Med 2012, 78:974-980.

3. Tan S, Li M, Ding X, et al. Effects of Fortunella margarita fruit extract on metabolic disorders in high-fat diet-induced obese C57BL/6 mice. PLoS One 2014, 9:e93510.

Leeks

1. Zhou Y, Zhuang W, Hu W, et al. Consumption of large amounts of Allium vegetables reduces risk for gastric cancer in a meta-analysis. Gastroenterology 2011, 141:80-89.

2. Galeone C, Pelucchi C, Levi F, et al. Onion and garlic use and human cancer. Am J Clin Nutr 2006, 84:1027-1032.

3. Guercio V, Turati F, La Vecchia C, et al. Allium vegetables and upper aerodigestive tract cancers: a meta-analysis of observational studies. Mol Nutr Food Res 2016, 60:212-222.

4. Casella S, Leonardi M, Melai B, et al. The role of diallyl sulfides and dipropyl sulfides in the in vitro antimicrobial activity of the essential oil of garlic, Allium sativum L., and leek, Allium porrum L. Phytother Res 2013, 27:380-383.

5. Fattorusso E, Lanzotti V, Taglialatela-Scafati O, Cicala C. The flavonoids of leek, Allium porrum. Phytochmistry 2001, 57:565-569.

6. Salvamani S, Gunasekaran B, Shaharuddin NA, et al. Antiartherosclerotic effects of plant flavonoids. Biomed Res Int 2014, 2014:480258.

Lentils

1. Bazzano LA, Thompson AM, Tees MT, et al. Non-soy legume consumption lowers cholesterol levels: a meta-analysis of randomized controlled trials. Nutrition, metabolism, and cardiovascular diseases : NMCD 2011, 21:94-103.

2. Mollard RC, Luhovyy BL, Panahi S, et al. Regular consumption of pulses for 8 weeks reduces metabolic syndrome risk factors in overweight and obese adults. Br J Nutr 2012, 108 Suppl 1:S111-122.

3. Mollard RC, Zykus A, Luhovyy BL, et al. The acute effects of a pulse-containing meal on glycaemic responses and measures of satiety and satiation within and at a later meal. Br J Nutr 2012, 108:509-517.

4. Ganesan K, Xu B. Polyphenol-Rich Lentils and Their Health Promoting Effects. Int J Mol Sci 2017, 18.

Lima Beans

1. Zhu B, Sun Y, Qi L, et al. Dietary legume consumption reduces risk of colorectal cancer: evidence from a meta-analysis of cohort studies. Sci Rep 2015, 5:8797.

2. Bazzano LA, Thompson AM, Tees MT, et al. Non-soy legume consumption lowers cholesterol levels: a meta-analysis of randomized controlled trials. Nutrition, metabolism, and cardiovascular diseases: NMCD 2011, 21:94-103.

3. Sievenpiper JL, Kendall CW, Esfahani A, et al. Effect of non-oil-seed pulses on glycaemic control: a systematic review and meta-analysis of randomised controlled experimental trials in people with and without diabetes. Diab tologia 2009, 52:1479-1495.

Mango

1. Burton-Freeman BM, Sandhu AK, Edirisinghe I. Mangos and their bioactive components: adding variety to the fruit plate for

health. Food Funct 2017, 8:3010-3032.

2. Evans SF, Meister M, Mahmood M, et al. Mango supplementation improves blood glucose in obese individuals. Nutr Metab Insights 2014, 7:77-84.

3. Noratto GD, Bertoldi MC, Krenek K, et al. Anticarcinogenic effects of polyphenolics from mango (Mangifera indica) varieties. J Agric Food Chem 2010, 58:4104-4112.

Melons (Cantaloupe, Honeydew)
1. Min KB, Min JY. Association between leukocyte telomere length and serum carotenoid in US adults. Eur J Nutr 2016.

Mixed Baby Greens
1. Roe LS, Meengs JS, Rolls BJ. Salad and satiety. The effect of timing of salad consumption on meal energy intake. Appetite 2012, 58:242-248.

2. Rolls BJ, Roe LS, Meengs JS. Salad and satiety: energy density and portion size of a first-course salad affect energy intake at lunch. J Am Diet Assoc 2004, 104:1570-1576.

3. Cox BD, Whichelow MJ, Prevost AT. Seasonal consumption of salad vegetables and fresh fruit in relation to the development of cardiovascular disease and cancer. Public Health Nutr 2000, 3:19-29.

4. WCRF/AICR Expert Report, Food, Nutrition, Physical Activity and the Prevention of Cancer: a Global Perspective. 2007 [dietandcancerreport.org]

5. Lockheart MS, Steffen LM, Rebnord HM, et al. Dietary patterns, food groups and myocardial infarction: a case-control study. Br J Nutr 2007, 98:380-387.

Mushrooms
1. Jeong SC, Koyyalamudi SR, Pang G. Dietary intake of Agaricus bisporus white button mushroom accelerates salivary immunoglobulin A secretion in healthy volunteers. Nutrition 2012, 28:527-531.

2. Ren L, Perera C, Hemar Y. Antitumor activity of mushroom polysaccharides: a review. Food Funct 2012, 3:1118-1130.

3. Chen S, Oh SR, Phung S, et al. Anti-aromatase activity of phytochemicals in white button mushrooms (Agaricus bisporus). Cancer Res 2006, 66:12026-12034.

4. Zhang M, Huang J, Xie X, Holman CD. Dietary intakes of mushrooms and green tea combine to reduce the risk of breast cancer in Chinese women. Int J Cancer 2009, 124:1404-1408.

5. Martin KR. Both common and specialty mushrooms inhibit adhesion molecule expression and in vitro binding of monocytes to human aortic endothelial cells in a pro-inflammatory environment. Nutr J 2010, 9:29.

6. Guillamon E, Garcia-Lafuente A, Lozano M, et al. Edible mushrooms: role in the prevention of cardiovascular diseases. Fitoterapia 2010, 81:715-723.

7. Schulzova V, Hajslova J, Peroutka R, et al. Influence of storage and household processing on the agaritine content of the cultivated Agaricus mushroom. Food Addit Contam 2002, 19:853-862.

Mustard and Turnip Greens
1. Higdon J, Drake VJ, Delage B. Linus Pauling Institute, Oregon State University. Micronutrient Information Center. Cruciferous Vegetables. In 2016 [http://lpi.oregonstate.edu/mic/food-beverages/cruciferous-vegetables]

2. Giordano P, Scicchitano P, Locorotondo M, et al. Carotenoids and cardiovascular risk. Curr Pharm Des 2012, 18:5577-5589.

3. Kopcke W, Krutmann J. Protection from sunburn with beta-Carotene--a meta-analysis. Photochem Photobiol 2008, 84:284-288.

4. Stahl W, Sies H. beta-Carotene and other carotenoids in protection from sunlight. Am J Clin Nutr 2012.

5. Stringham JM, Bovier ER, Wong JC, Hammond BR, Jr. The influence of dietary lutein and zeaxanthin on visual performance. J Food Sci 2010, 75:R24-29.

Nectarines
1. McCullough ML, Peterson JJ, Patel R, et al. Flavonoid intake and cardiovascular disease mortality in a prospective cohort of US adults. Am J Clin Nutr 2012.

2. Wang X, Ouyang YY, Liu J, Zhao G. Flavonoid intake and risk of CVD: a systematic review and meta-analysis of prospective cohort studies. Br J Nutr 2014, 111:1-11.

3. Redondo D, Arias E, Oria R, Venturini ME. Thinned stone fruits are a source of polyphenols and antioxidant compounds. J Sci Food Agric 2017, 97:902-910.

4. Cires MJ, Wong X, Carrasco-Pozo C, Gotteland M. The Gastrointestinal Tract as a Key Target Organ for the Health-Promoting Effects of Dietary Proanthocyanidins. Front Nutr 2016, 3:57.

5. Nandakumar V, Singh T, Katiyar SK. Multi-targeted prevention and therapy of cancer by proanthocyanidins. Cancer Lett 2008, 269:378-387.

Okra
1. Brown L, Rosner B, Willett WW, Sacks FM. Cholesterol-lowering effects of dietary fiber: a meta-analysis. Am J Clin Nutr 1999, 69:30-42.

Onions
1. Galeone C, Pelucchi C, Levi F, et al. Onion and garlic use and human cancer. Am J Clin Nutr 2006, 84:1027-1032.

2. Slimestad R, Fossen T, Vagen IM. Onions: a source of unique dietary flavonoids. J Agric Food Chem 2007, 55:10067-10080.

3. Ravasco P, Aranha MM, Borralho PM, et al. Colorectal cancer: can nutrients modulate NF-kappaB and apoptosis? Clin Nutr 2010, 29:42-46.

4. Miyamoto S, Yasui Y, Ohigashi H, et al. Dietary flavonoids suppress azoxymethane-induced colonic preneoplastic lesions in male C57BL/KsJ-db/db mice. Chem Biol Interact 2010, 183:276-283.

5. Shan BE, Wang MX, Li RQ. Quercetin inhibit human SW480 colon cancer growth in association with inhibition of cyclin D1 and survivin expression through Wnt/beta-catenin signaling pathway. Cancer Invest 2009, 27:604-612.

6. Pierini R, Gee JM, Belshaw NJ, Johnson IT. Flavonoids and intestinal cancers. Br J Nutr 2008, 99 E Suppl 1:ES53-59.

7. Powolny A, Singh S. Multitargeted prevention and therapy of cancer by diallyl trisulfide and related Allium vegetable-derived organosulfur compounds. Cancer Lett 2008, 269:305-314.

Orange
1. Testai L, Calderone V. Nutraceutical Value of Citrus Flavanones and Their Implications in Cardiovascular Disease. Nutrients 2017, 9.

Papaya
1. Schweiggert RM, Kopec RE, Villalobos-Gutierrez MG, et al. Carotenoids are more bioavailable from papaya than from tomato and carrot in humans: a randomised cross-over study. Br J Nutr 2014, 111:490-498.

2. Pandey VP, Dwivedi UN. A ripening associated peroxidase from papaya having a role in defense and lignification: heterologous expression and in-silico and in-vitro experimental validation. Gene 2015, 555:438-447.

3. Somanah J, Bourdon E, Bahorun T. Extracts of Mauritian Carica papaya (var. solo) protect SW872 and HepG2 cells against hydrogen peroxide induced oxidative stress. J Food Sci Technol 2017, 54:1917-1927.

4. Somanah J, Aruoma OI, Gunness TK, et al. Effects of a short term supplementation of a fermented papaya preparation on biomarkers of diabetes mellitus in a randomized Mauritian population. Prev Med 2012, 54 Suppl:S90-97.

Parsnips
1. Brown L, Rosner B, Willett WW, Sacks FM. Cholesterol-lowering effects of dietary fiber: a meta-analysis. Am J Clin Nutr 1999, 69:30-42.

2. Higdon J, Drake VJ: Fiber. In An Evidence-based Approach to Phytochemicals and Other Dietary Factors New York: Thieme; 2013: 133-148

Peaches
1. Noratto G, Porter W, Byrne D, Cisneros-Zevallos L. Identifying peach and plum polyphenols with chemopreventive potential against estrogen-independent breast cancer cells. J Agric Food Chem 2009, 57:5219-5226.

Pears
1. Reiland H, Slavin J. Systematic Review of Pears and Health. Nutr Today 2015, 50:301-305.

2. Oude Griep LM, Verschuren WM, Kromhout D, Ocke MC, Geleijnse JM. Colors of fruit and vegetables and 10-year incidence of stroke. Stroke 2011; 42:3190-3195.

3. Streppel MT, Arends LR, van 't Veer P, et al. Dietary fiber and blood pressure: a meta-analysis of randomized placebo-controlled trials. Arch Intern Med 2005, 165:150-156.

4. Marunaka Y, Marunaka R, Sun H, et al. Actions of Quercetin, a Polyphenol, on Blood Pressure. Molecules 2017, 22.

Peas (Green, Split, Sugar Snap, Snow)
1. Hernandez-Ramirez RU, Galvan-Portillo MV, Ward MH, et al. Dietary intake of polyphenols, nitrate and nitrite and gastric cancer risk in Mexico City. Int J Cancer 2009, 125:1424-1430.

2. Zafar A, Singh S, Satija YK, et al. Deciphering the molecular mechanism underlying anticancer activity of coumestrol in triple-negative breast cancer cells. Toxicol In Vitro 2018, 46:19-28.

3. Hedelin M, Lof M, Olsson M, et al. Dietary phytoestrogens are not associated with risk of overall breast cancer but diets rich in coumestrol are inversely associated with risk of estrogen receptor and progesterone receptor negative breast tumors in Swedish women. J Nutr 2008, 138:938-945.

4. de Kleijn MJ, van der Schouw YT, Wilson PW, et al. Intake of dietary phytoestrogens is low in postmenopausal women in the United States: the Framingham study(1-4). J Nutr 2001, 131:1826-1832.

5. Hwang YW, Kim SY, Jee SH, et al. Soy food consumption and risk of prostate cancer: a meta-analysis of observational studies. Nutr Cancer 2009, 61:598-606.

6. Trock BJ, Hilakivi-Clarke L, Clarke R. Meta-analysis of soy intake and breast cancer risk. J Natl Cancer Inst 2006, 98:459-471.

7. Fritz H, Seely D, Flower G, et al. Soy, red clover, and isoflavones and breast cancer: a systematic review. PLoS One 2013, 8:e81968.

8. Wu AH, Yu MC, Tseng CC, Pike MC. Epidemiology of soy exposures and breast cancer risk. Br J Cancer 2008, 98:9-14.

9. Darmadi-Blackberry I, Wahlqvist ML, Kouris-Blazos A, et al. Legumes: the most important dietary predictor of survival in older people of different ethnicities. Asia Pac J Clin Nutr 2004, 13:217-220.

10. Hosseinpour-Niazi S, Mirmiran P, Amiri Z, et al. Legume intake is inversely associated with metabolic syndrome in adults. Arch Iran Med 2012, 15:538-544.

11. Bazzano LA, Thompson AM, Tees MT, et al. Non-soy legume consumption lowers cholesterol levels: a meta-analysis of randomized controlled trials. Nutrition, metabolism, and cardiovascular diseases : NMCD 2011, 21:94-103.

12. Marventano S, Izquierdo Pulido M, Sanchez-Gonzalez C, et al. Legume consumption and CVD risk: a systematic review and meta-analysis. Public Health Nutr 2017, 20:245-254.

13. Zhu B, Sun Y, Qi L, et al. Dietary legume consumption reduces risk of colorectal cancer: evidence from a meta-analysis of cohort studies. Sci Rep 2015, 5:8797.

Pecans

1. Bolling BW, Chen CY, McKay DL, Blumberg JB. Tree nut phytochemicals: composition, antioxidant capacity, bioactivity, impact factors. A systematic review of almonds, Brazils, cashews, hazelnuts, macadamias, pecans, pine nuts, pistachios and walnuts. Nutr Res Rev 2011:1-32.

2. Hudthagosol C, Haddad EH, McCarthy K, et al. Pecans Acutely Increase Plasma Postprandial Antioxidant Capacity and Catechins and Decrease LDL Oxidation in Humans. J Nutr 2011, 141:56-62.

3. Morgan WA, Clayshulte BJ. Pecans lower low-density lipoprotein cholesterol in people with normal lipid levels. J Am Diet Assoc 2000, 100:312-318.

4. Kris-Etherton PM, Hu FB, Ros E, Sabate J. The role of tree nuts and peanuts in the prevention of coronary heart disease: multiple potential mechanisms. J Nutr 2008, 138:1746S-1751S.

5. Grosso G, Yang J, Marventano S, et al. Nut consumption on all-cause, cardiovascular, and cancer mortality risk: a systematic review and meta-analysis of epidemiologic studies. Am J Clin Nutr 2015, 101:783-793.

Peppers (Bell)

1. Fernandez-Garcia E, Carvajal-Lerida I, Perez-Galvez A. Carotenoids exclusively synthesized in red pepper (capsanthin and capsorubin) protect human dermal fibroblasts against UVB induced DNA damage. Photochem Photobiol Sci 2016, 15:1204-1211.

2. Tian SL, Li L, Chai WG, et al. Effects of silencing key genes in the capsanthin biosynthetic pathway on fruit color of detached pepper fruits. BMC Plant Biol 2014, 14:314.

3. Lin Y, Shi R, Wang X, Shen HM. Luteolin, a flavonoid with potential for cancer prevention and therapy. Curr Cancer Drug Targets 2008, 8:634-646.

4. Bartke A. Minireview: role of the growth hormone/insulin-like growth factor system in mammalian aging. Endocrinology 2005, 146:3718-3723.

5. Lim DY, Cho HJ, Kim J, et al. Luteolin decreases IGF-II production and downregulates insulin-like growth factor-I receptor signaling in HT-29 human colon cancer cells. BMC Gastroenterol 2012, 12:9.

Pineapple

1. Pavan R, Jain S, Shraddha, Kumar A. Properties and therapeutic application of bromelain: a review. Biotechnol Res Int 2012, 2012:976203.

2. Chobotova K, Vernallis AB, Majid FA. Bromelain's activity and potential as an anti-cancer agent: Current evidence and perspectives. Cancer Lett 2010, 290:148-156.

3. Wang L, Tang DQ, Kuang Y, et al. Structural characteristics of pineapple pulp polysaccharides and their antitumor cell proliferation activities. J Sci Food Agric 2015, 95:2554-2561.

4. Izquierdo-Vega JA, Morales-Gonzalez JA, SanchezGutierrez M, et al. Evidence of Some Natural Products with Antigenotoxic Effects. Part 1: Fruits and Polysaccharides. Nutrients 2017, 9.

5. Linus Pauling Institue Micronutrient Information Center. Manganese [http://lpi.oregonstate.edu/infocenter/minerals/manganese/]

Pine Nuts

1. Wolff RL, Pedrono F, Pasquier E, Marpeau AM. General characteristics of Pinus spp. seed fatty acid compositions, and importance of delta5-olefinic acids in the taxonomy and phylogeny of the genus. Lipids 2000, 35:1-22.

2. Pasman WJ, Heimerikx J, Rubingh CM, et al. The effect of Korean pine nut oil on in vitro CCK release, on appetite sensations and on gut hormones in post-menopausal overweight women. Lipids in Health and Disease 2008, 7:10.

3. Nasri N, Fady B, Triki S. Quantification of sterols and aliphatic alcohols in Mediterranean stone pine (Pinus pinea L.) populations. Journal of agricultural and food chemistry 2007, 55:2251-2255.

4. NutritionData.com: Nutrient Search Tool [http://www.nutritiondata.com/tools/nutrient-search]

5. Berger A, Jones PJ, Abumweis SS. Plant sterols: factors affecting their efficacy and safety as functional food ingredients. Lipids Health Dis 2004, 3:5.

6. Woyengo TA, Ramprasath VR, Jones PJ. Anticancer effects of phytosterols. Eur J Clin Nutr 2009, 63:813-820.

7. Mendilaharsu M, De Stefani E, Deneo-Pellegrini H, et al. Phytosterols and risk of lung cancer: a case-control study in Uruguay. Lung Cancer 1998, 21:37-45.

8. Ronco A, De Stefani E, Boffetta P, et al. Vegetables, fruits, and related nutrients and risk of breast cancer: a case-control study in Uruguay. Nutr Cancer 1999, 35:111-119.

9. De Stefani E, Brennan P, Boffetta P, et al. Vegetables, fruits, related dietary antioxidants, and risk of squamous cell carcinoma of the esophagus: a case-control study in Uruguay. Nutr Cancer 2000, 38:23-29.

10. De Stefani E, Boffetta P, Ronco AL, et al. Plant sterols and risk of stomach cancer: a case-control study in Uruguay. Nutr Cancer 2000, 37:140-144.

Pistachios

1. Ellegard LH, Andersson SW, Normen AL, Andersson HA. Dietary plant sterols and cholesterol metabolism. Nutr Rev 2007, 65:39-45.

2. Kay CD, Gebauer SK, West SG, Kris-Etherton PM. Pistachios increase serum antioxidants and lower serum oxidized-LDL in hypercholesterolemic adults. J Nutr 2010, 140:1093-1098.

3. Kocyigit A, Koylu AA, Keles H. Effects of pistachio nuts consumption on plasma lipid profile and oxidative status in healthy volunteers. Nutrition, metabolism, and cardiovascular diseases : NMCD 2006, 16:202-209.

4. Sari I, Baltaci Y, Bagci C, et al. Effect of pistachio diet on lipid parameters, endothelial function, inflammation, and oxidative status: a prospective study. Nutrition 2010, 26:399-404.

5. Aldemir M, Okulu E, Neselioglu S, et al. Pistachio diet improves erectile function parameters and serum lipid profiles in patients with erectile dysfunction. Int J Impot Res 2011, 23:32-38.

Plums

1. Lever E, Cole J, Scott SM, et al. Systematic review: the effect of prunes on gastrointestinal function. Aliment Pharmacol Ther 2014, 40:750-758.

2. Arjmandi BH, Johnson SA, Pourafshar S, et al. Bone-Protective Effects of Dried Plum in Postmenopausal Women: Efficacy and Possible Mechanisms. Nutrients 2017, 9.

Pomegranate

1. Howell AB, D'Souza DH. The pomegranate: effects on bacteria and viruses that influence human health. Evid Based Complement Alternat Med 2013, 2013:606212.

2. Aviram M, Dornfeld L, Rosenblat M, et al. Pomegranate juice consumption reduces oxidative stress, atherogenic modifications to LDL, and platelet aggregation: studies in humans and in atherosclerotic apolipoprotein E-deficient mice. Am J Clin Nutr 2000, 71:1062-1076.

3. Adhami VM, Khan N, Mukhtar H. Cancer chemoprevention by pomegranate: laboratory and clinical evidence. Nutr Cancer 2009, 61:811-815.

4. Pantuck AJ, Leppert JT, Zomorodian N, et al. Phase II study of pomegranate juice for men with rising prostate-specific antigen following surgery or radiation for prostate cancer. Clin Cancer Res 2006, 12:4018-4026.

5. Paller CJ, Ye X, Wozniak PJ, et al. A randomized phase II study of pomegranate extract for men with rising PSA following initial therapy for localized prostate cancer. Prostate Cancer Prostatic Dis 2013, 16:50-55.

6. Aviram M, Rosenblat M, Gaitini D, et al. Pomegranate juice consumption for 3 years by patients with carotid artery stenosis reduces common carotid intima-media thickness, blood pressure and LDL oxidation. Clin Nutr 2004, 23:423-433.

7. Bookheimer SY, Renner BA, Ekstrom A, et al. Pomegranate juice augments memory and FMRI activity in middle-aged and older adults with mild memory complaints. Evid Based Complement Alternat Med 2013, 2013:946298.

Pumpkin

1. Shardell MD, Alley DE, Hicks GE, et al. Low-serum carotenoid concentrations and carotenoid interactions predict mortality in US adults: the Third National Health and Nutrition Examination Survey. Nutr Res 2011, 31:178-189.

2. Min KB, Min JY. Association between leukocyte telomere length and serum carotenoid in US adults. Eur J Nutr 2016.

3. Oregon State University. Linus Pauling Institute Micronutrient Information Center. Vitamin A. In [http://lpi.oregonstate.edu/infocenter/vitamins/vitaminA/]

Pumpkin Seeds

1. King JC. Zinc: an essential but elusive nutrient. Am J Clin Nutr 2011, 94:679S-684S.

2. Prasad AS. Zinc in human health: effect of zinc on immune cells. Mol Med 2008, 14:353-357.

3. Barnett JB, Hamer DH, Meydani SN. Low zinc status: a new risk factor for pneumonia in the elderly? Nutr Rev 2010, 68:30-37.

4. Office of Dietary Supplements, National Institutes of Health. Dietary Supplement Fact Sheet: Zinc. [http://ods.od.nih.gov/factsheets/Zinc-HealthProfessional/]

5. Mocchegiani E, Romeo J, Malavolta M, et al. Zinc: dietary intake and impact of supplementation on immune function in elderly. Age (Dordr) 2013, 35:839-860.

Quinoa

1. Office of Dietary Supplements, National Institutes of Health. Magnesium. 2016.

2. Graf BL, Rojas-Silva P, Rojo LE, et al. Innovations in Health Value and Functional Food Development of Quinoa (Chenopodium quinoa Willd.). Compr Rev Food Sci Food Saf 2015, 14:431-445.

3. Tang Y, Tsao R. Phytochemicals in quinoa and amaranth grains and their antioxidant, anti-inflammatory, and potential health beneficial effects: a review. Mol Nutr Food Res 2017, 61.

Radicchio

1. D'Evoli L, Morroni F, Lombardi-Boccia G, et al. Red chicory (Cichorium intybus L. cultivar) as a potential source of antioxidant anthocyanins for intestinal health. Oxid Med Cell Longev 2013, 2013:704310.

2. Azzini E, Maiani G, Garaguso I, et al. The Potential Health Benefits of Polyphenol-Rich Extracts from Cichorium intybus L. Studied on Caco-2 Cells Model. Oxid Med Cell Longev 2016, 2016:1594616.

Radishes

1. Yang M, Wang H, Zhou M, et al. The natural compound sulforaphene, as a novel anticancer reagent, targeting PI3K-AKT signaling pathway in lung cancer. Oncotarget 2016, 7:76656-76666.

2. Pawlik A, Wala M, Hac A, et al. Sulforaphene, an isothiocyanate present in radish plants, inhibits proliferation of human breast cancer cells. Phytomedicine 2017, 29:1-10.

3. Beevi SS, Mangamoori LN, Subathra M, Edula JR. Hexane extract of Raphanus sativus L. roots inhibits cell proliferation and induces apoptosis in human cancer cells by modulating

genes related to apoptotic pathway. Plant Foods Hum Nutr 2010, 65:200-209.

Raspberries

1. Burton-Freeman BM, Sandhu AK, Edirisinghe I. Red Raspberries and Their Bioactive Polyphenols: Cardiometabolic and Neuronal Health Links. Adv Nutr 2016, 7:44-65.

2. Mallery SR, Tong M, Shumway BS, et al. Topical application of a mucoadhesive freeze-dried black raspberry gel induces clinical and histologic regression and reduces loss of heterozygosity events in premalignant oral intraepithelial lesions: results from a multicentered, placebo-controlled clinical trial. Clin Cancer Res 2014, 20:1910-1924.

3. Mentor-Marcel RA, Bobe G, Sardo C, et al. Plasma cytokines as potential response indicators to dietary freeze-dried black raspberries in colorectal cancer patients. Nutr Cancer 2012, 64:820-825.

Romaine

1. Office of Dietary Supplements, National Institutes of Health. Dietary Supplement Fact Sheet: Folate [http://ods.od.nih.gov/factsheets/Folate-HealthProfessional/]

2. Linus Pauling Institute, Oregon State University. Micronutrient Information Center: Folate. In 2014 [http://lpi.oregonstate.edu/mic/vitamins/folate]

3. Baggott JE, Oster RA, Tamura T. Meta-analysis of cancer risk in folic acid supplementation trials. Cancer Epidemiol 2011.

Rutabaga

1. Pasko P, Bukowska-Strakova K, Gdula-Argasinska J, Tyszka-Czochara M. Rutabaga (Brassica napus L. var. napobrassica) seeds, roots, and sprouts: a novel kind of food with antioxidant properties and proapoptotic potential in Hep G2 hepatoma cell line. J Med Food 2013, 16:749-759.

Scallions

1. Powolny A, Singh S. Multitargeted prevention and therapy of cancer by diallyl trisulfide and related Allium vegetable-derived organosulfur compounds. Cancer Lett 2008; 269:305-314.

Sesame Seeds

1. Higdon J: Lignans. In An Evidence-Based Approach to Dietary Phytochemicals. New York: Thieme; 2006: 155-161

Spinach

1. Clements WT, Lee SR, Bloomer RJ. Nitrate ingestion: a review of the health and physical performance effects. Nutrients 2014, 6:5224-5264.

2. Lara J, Ashor AW, Oggioni C, et al. Effects of inorganic nitrate and beetroot supplementation on endothelial function: a systematic review and meta-analysis. Eur J Nutr 2016, 55:451-459.

3. Jovanovski E, Bosco L, Khan K, et al. Effect of Spinach, a High Dietary Nitrate Source, on Arterial Stiffness and Related Hemodynamic Measures: A Randomized, Controlled Trial in Healthy Adults. Clin Nutr Res 2015, 4:160-167.

4. Office of Dietary Supplements, National Institutes of Health. Magnesium. 2016.

5. Weaver CM, Proulx WR, Heaney R. Choices for achieving adequate dietary calcium with a vegetarian diet. Am J Clin Nutr 1999, 70:543S-548S.

Strawberries

1. Mink PJ, Scrafford CG, Barraj LM, et al. Flavonoid intake and cardiovascular disease mortality: a prospective study in postmenopausal women. Am J Clin Nutr 2007, 85:895-909.

2. Basu A, Lyons TJ. Strawberries, Blueberries, and Cranberries in the Metabolic Syndrome: Clinical Perspectives. Journal of Agricultural and Food Chemis ry 2011.

3. Zunino SJ, Parelman MA, Freytag TL, et al. Effects of dietary strawberry powder on blood lipids and inflammatory markers in obese human subjects. Br J Nutr 2011:1-10.

4. Basu A, Wilkinson M, Penugonda K, et al. Freeze-dried strawberry powder improves lipid profile and lipid peroxidation in women with metabolic syndrome: baseline and post intervention effects. Nutr J 2009, 8:43.

5. Basu A, Betts NM, Nguyen A, et al. Freeze-dried strawberries lower serum cholesterol and lipid peroxidation in adults with abdominal adiposity and elevated serum lipids. J Nutr 2014, 144:830-837.

6. Edirisinghe I, Banaszewski K, Cappozzo J, et al. Strawberry anthocyanin and its association with postprandial inflammation and insulin. Br J Nutr 2011, 106:913-922.

7. Basu A, Fu DX, Wilkinson M, et al. Strawberries decrease atherosclerotic markers in subjects with metabolic syndrome. Nutr Res 2010, 30:462-469.

8. Moazen S, Amani R, Homayouni Rad A, et al. Effects of freeze-dried strawberry supplementation on metabolic biomarkers of atherosclerosis in subjects with type 2 diabetes: a randomized double-blind controlled trial. Ann Nutr Metab 2013, 63:256-264.

9. Burton-Freeman B, Linares A, Hyson D, Kappagoda T. Strawberry modulates LDL oxidation and postprandial lipemia in response to high-fat meal in overweight hyperlipidemic men and women. J Am Coll Nutr 2010, 29:46-54.

10. Jenkins DJ, Nguyen TH, Kendall CW, et al. The effect of strawberries in a cholesterol-lowering dietary portfolio. Metabolism 2008, 57:1636-1644.

11. Park E, Edirisinghe I, Wei H, et al. A dose-response evaluation of freeze-dried strawberries independent of fiber content on metabolic indices in abdominally obese individuals with insulin resistance in a randomized, single-blinded, diet-controlled crossover trial. Mol Nutr Food Res 2016, 60:1099-1109.

12. Chen T, Yan F, Qian J, et al. Randomized phase II trial of lyophilized strawberries in patients with dysplastic precancerous lesions of the esophagus. Cancer Prev Res (Phila) 2012, 5:41-50.

Sunflower Seeds

1. Bjelakovic G, Nikolova D, Gluud C. Meta-regression analyses, meta-analyses, and trial sequential analyses of the effects of

supplementation with beta-carotene, vitamin A, and vitamin E singly or in different combinations on all-cause mortality: do we have evidence for lack of harm? PLoS One 2013, 8:e74558.

2. Mathur P, Ding Z, Saldeen T, Mehta JL. Tocopherols in the Prevention and Treatment of Atherosclerosis and Related Cardiovascular Disease. Clin Cardiol 2015, 38:570-576.

3. Phillips KM, Ruggio DM, Ashraf-Khorassani M. Phytosterol composition of nuts and seeds commonly consumed in the United States. J Agric Food Chem 2005, 53:9436-9445.

Sweet Potatoes

1. Oregon State University. Linus Pauling Institute Micronutrient Information Center. Vitamin A. In [http://lpi.oregonstate.edu/infocenter/vitamins/vitaminA/]

2. van Leeuwen R, Boekhoorn S, Vingerling JR, et al. Dietary intake of antioxidants and risk of age-related macular degeneration. JAMA 2005, 294:3101-3107.

3. Evans JA, Johnson EJ. The role of phytonutrients in skin health. Nutrients 2010, 2:903-928.

4. Kopcke W, Krutmann J. Protection from sunburn with beta-Carotene--a meta-analysis. Photochem Photobiol 2008, 84:284-288.

Swiss chard

1. Stringham JM, Bovier ER, Wong JC, Hammond BR, Jr. The influence of dietary lutein and zeaxanthin on visual performance. J Food Sci 2010, 75:R24-29.

2. Clifford T, Howatson G, West DJ, Stevenson EJ. The potential benefits of red beetroot supplementation in health and disease. Nutrients 2015, 7:2801-2822.

Tomatoes

1. van het Hof KH, de Boer BC, Tijburg LB, et al. Carotenoid bioavailability in humans from tomatoes processed in different ways determined from the carotenoid response in the triglyceride-rich lipoprotein fraction of plasma after a single consumption and in plasma after four days of consumption. J Nutr 2000, 130:1189-1196.

2. USDA National Nutrient Database for Standard Reference [http://ndb.nal.usda.gov/ndb/search/list]

3. Rizwan M, Rodriguez-Blanco I, Harbottle A, et al. Tomato paste rich in lycopene protects against cutaneous photodamage in humans in vivo. Br J Dermatol 2010.

4. Palozza P, Parrone N, Catalano A, Simone R. Tomato lycopene and inflammatory cascade: basic interactions and clinical implications. Curr Med Chem 2010, 17:2547-2563.

5. Ried K, Fakler P. Protective effect of lycopene on serum cholesterol and blood pressure: Meta-analyses of intervention trials. Maturitas 2011, 68:299-310.

6. van Breemen RB, Pajkovic N. Multitargeted therapy of cancer by lycopene. Cancer Lett 2008, 269:339-351.

7. Karppi J, Laukkanen JA, Sivenius J, et al. Serum lycopene decreases the risk of stroke in men: A population-based follow-up study. Neurology 2012, 79:1540-1547.

8. Karppi J, Laukkanen JA, Makikallio TH, Kurl S. Low serum lycopene and beta-carotene increase risk of acute myocardial infarction in men. Eur J Public Health 2011.

9. Hak AE, Ma J, Powell CB, et al. Prospective study of plasma carotenoids and tocopherols in relation to risk of ischemic stroke. Stroke 2004, 35:1584-1588.

10. Sahni S, Hannan MT, Blumberg J, et al. Protective effect of total carotenoid and lycopene intake on the risk of hip fracture: a 17-year follow-up from the Framingham Osteoporosis Study. J Bone Miner Res 2009, 24:1086-1094.

Turmeric

1. Singh S, Aggarwal BB. Activation of transcription factor NF-kappa B is suppressed by curcumin (diferuloylmethane) [corrected]. J Biol Chem 1995, 270:24995-25000.

2. Sahebkar A. Are curcuminoids effective C-reactive protein-lowering agents in clinical practice? Evidence from a meta-analysis. Phytother Res 2014, 28:633-642.

3. Aggarwal BB, Yuan W, Li S, Gupta SC. Curcumin-free turmeric exhibits anti-inflammatory and anticancer activities: Identification of novel components of turmeric. Mol Nutr Food Res 2013, 57:1529-1542.

4. Park W, Amin AR, Chen ZG, Shin DM. New perspectives of curcumin in cancer prevention. Cancer Prev Res (Phila) 2013, 6:387-400.

5. Sandur SK, Pandey MK, Sung B, et al. Curcumin, demethoxy-curcumin, bisdemethoxycurcumin, tetrahydrocurcumin and turmerones differentially regulate anti-inflammatory and anti-proliferative responses through a ROS-independent mechanism. Carcinogenesis 2007, 28:1765-1773.

6. Panahi Y, Alishiri GH, Parvin S, Sahebkar A. Mitigation of Systemic Oxidative Stress by Curcuminoids in Osteoarthritis: Results of a Randomized Controlled Trial. J Diet Suppl 2016, 13:209-220.

7. Daily JW, Yang M, Park S. Efficacy of Turmeric Extracts and Curcumin for Alleviating the Symptoms of Joint Arthritis: A Systematic Review and Meta-Analysis of Randomized Clinical Trials. J Med Food 2016, 19:717-729.

8. Vaughn AR, Haas KN, Burney W, et al. Potential Role of Curcumin Against Biofilm-Producing Organisms on the Skin: A Review. Phytother Res 2017, 31:1807-1816.

Turnips

1. Higdon J, Drake VJ, Delage B. Linus Pauling Institute, Oregon State University. Micronutrient Information Center. Cruciferous Vegetables. In 2016 [http://lpi.oregonstate.edu/mic/food-beverages/cruciferous-vegetables]

Walnuts

1. Valls-Pedret C, Lamuela-Raventos RM, Medina-Remon A, et al. Polyphenol-rich foods in the Mediterranean diet are associated with better cognitive function in elderly subjects at high cardiovascular risk. J Alzheimers Dis 2012, 29:773-782.

2. Pribis P, Shukitt-Hale B. Cognition: the new frontier for nuts and berries. Am J Clin Nutr 2014, 100 Suppl 1:347S-352S.

3. Poulose SM, Miller MG, Shukitt-Hale B. Role of walnuts in maintaining brain health with age. J Nutr 2014, 144:561S-566S.

4. Higdon J, Drake VJ: Essential Fatty Acids. In An Evidence-Based Approach to Dietary Phytochemicals and Other Dietary Factors. Second edition. New York: Thieme; 2013: 183-208

5. Anderson KJ, Teuber SS, Gobeille A, et al. Walnut polyphenolics inhibit in vitro human plasma and LDL oxidation. J Nutr 2001, 131:2837-2842.

6. Sanchez-Gonzalez C, Ciudad CJ, Noe V, Izquierdo-Pulido M. Health benefits of walnut polyphenols: An exploration beyond their lipid profile. Crit Rev Food Sci Nutr 2017, 57:3373-3383.

7. Kris-Etherton PM. Walnuts decrease risk of cardiovascular disease: a summary of efficacy and biologic mechanisms. J Nutr 2014, 144:547S-554S.

8. Grosso G, Yang J, Marventano S, et al. Nut consumption on all-cause, cardiovascular, and cancer mortality risk: a systematic review and meta-analysis of epidemiologic studies. Am J Clin Nutr 2015, 101:783-793.

9. Ma Y, Njike VY, Millet J, et al. Effects of walnut consumption on endothelial function in type 2 diabetic subjects: a randomized controlled crossover trial. Diabetes Care 2010, 33:227-232.

10. Mattes RD, Dreher ML. Nuts and healthy body weight maintenance mechanisms. Asia Pac J Clin Nutr 2010, 19:137-141.

Watercress

1. Abdel-Aal el SM, Akhtar H, Zaheer K, Ali R. Dietary sources of lutein and zeaxanthin carotenoids and their role in eye health. Nutrients 2013, 5:1169-1185.

2. Hyun H, Park H, Jeong J, et al. Effects of Watercress Containing Rutin and Rutin Alone on the Proliferation and Osteogenic Differentiation of Human Osteoblast-like MG-63 Cells. Korean J Physiol Pharmacol 2014, 18:347-352.

3. Syed Alwi SS, Cavell BE, Telang U, et al. In vivo modulation of 4E binding protein 1 (4E-BP1) phosphorylation by watercress: a pilot study. Br J Nutr 2010:1-9.

4. Watercress may 'turn off' breast cancer signal [http://www.soton.ac.uk/mediacentre/news/2010/sep/10_94.shtml]

5. Fogarty MC, Hughes CM, Burke G, et al. Acute and chronic watercress supplementation attenuates exercise-induced peripheral mononuclear cell DNA damage and lipid peroxidation. Br J Nutr 2013, 109:293-301.

Watermelon

1. Figueroa A, Sanchez-Gonzalez MA, Perkins-Veazie PM, Arjmandi BH. Effects of watermelon supplementation on aortic blood pressure and wave reflection in individuals with prehypertension: a pilot study. Am J Hypertens 2011, 24:40-44.

2. Figueroa A, Sanchez-Gonzalez MA, Wong A, Arjmandi BH. Watermelon extract supplementation reduces ankle blood pressure and carotid augmentation index in obese adults with prehypertension or hypertension. Am J Hypertens 2012, 25:640-643.

3. Edwards AJ, Vinyard BT, Wiley ER, et al. Consumption of watermelon juice increases plasma concentrations of lycopene and beta-carotene in humans. J Nutr 2003, 133:1043-1050.

4. Rissanen TH, Voutilainen S, Nyyssonen K, et al. Low serum lycopene concentration is associated with an excess incidence of acute coronary events and stroke: the Kuopio Ischaemic Heart Disease Risk Factor Study. Br J Nutr 2001, 85:749-754.

5. Rissanen T, Voutilainen S, Nyyssonen K, Salonen JT. Lycopene, atherosclerosis, and coronary heart disease. Exp Biol Med (Maywood) 2002, 227:900-907.

6. Rissanen TH, Voutilainen S, Nyyssonen K, et al. Serum lycopene concentrations and carotid atherosclerosis: the Kuopio Ischaemic Heart Disease Risk Factor Study. Am J Clin Nutr 2003, 77:133-138.

7. Hak AE, Ma J, Powell CB, et al. Prospective study of plasma carotenoids and tocopherols in relation to risk of ischemic stroke. Stroke 2004, 35:1584-1588.

8. Tarazona-Diaz MP, Alacid F, Carrasco M, et al. Watermelon juice: potential functional drink for sore muscle relief in athletes. J Agric Food Chem 2013, 61:7522-7528.

Winter Squash

1. Evans JA, Johnson EJ. The role of phytonutrients in skin health. Nutrients 2010, 2:903-928.

2. Stahl W, Sies H. beta-Carotene and other carotenoids in protection from sunlight. Am J Clin Nutr 2012.

3. Shardell MD, Alley DE, Hicks GE, et al. Low-serum carotenoid concentrations and carotenoid interactions predict mortality in US adults: the Third National Health and Nutrition Examination Survey. Nutr Res 2011, 31:178-189.

Zucchini

1. Lust TA, Paris HS. Italian horticultural and culinary records of summer squash (Cucurbita pepo, Cucurbitaceae) and emergence of the zucchini in 19th-century Milan. Ann Bot 2016, 118:503-69.

2. Zhang Z, Cogswell ME, Gillespie C, et al. Association between usual sodium and potassium intake and blood pressure and hypertension among U.S. adults: NHANES 2005-2010. PLoS One 2013, 8:e75289.

3. Oregon State University. Linus Pauling Institute. Micronutrient Information Center. Carotenoids. In 2016 [http://lpi.oregonstate.edu/mic/dietary-factors/phytochemicals/carotenoids]